Yoga with Weights

FOR

DUMMIES®

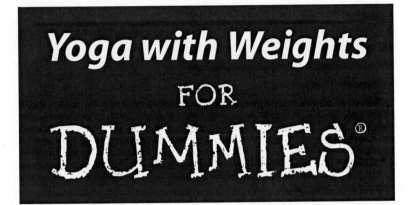

by Sherri Baptiste with Megan Scott, PhD

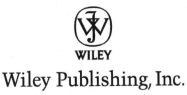

WILEY

Wiley Publishing, Inc.

Yoga with Weights For Dummies®
Published by
Wiley Publishing, Inc.
111 River St.
Hoboken, NJ 07030-5774
www.wiley.com

WILEY

About the Authors

Sherri Baptiste is an inspirational teacher at the forefront of yoga training in the United States. She was born into a rich heritage and family of pioneering teachers; her parents, Magaña and Walt Baptiste, established yoga on the West Coast in the mid-1950s. Her brother, Baron Baptiste, authored the book *Journey into Power: How to Sculpt Your Ideal Body, Free Your True Self, and Transform Your Life With Yoga* (Fireside). Sherri has been teaching yoga since her teens and is the founder of "Baptiste Power of Yoga," a nationally recognized yoga method, as well as a yoga-with-weights teacher-training program and a yoga teacher certification and advancing studies program recognized by *Yoga Alliance*. Sherri presents classes and workshops throughout the United States; she's a presenter for Western Athletics' Bay Clubs, Gold's Gym, Nautilus, Equinox, IDEA World Fitness, Body Mind Spirit, ECA; and she offers many yoga retreats, including retreats at Kripalu, Omega, Haramara, Green Gulch Zen Center, Rancho La Puerta Spa, and Feathered Pipe Ranch. A radio and television personality, she's featured in video, DVD, and CD "Power of Yoga" and "Power of Meditation" programs. You can learn more about Sherri at the following Web sites: www.powerofyoga.com and www.yogawithweights.com.

Megan Scott, PhD, is a doctor of integrative medicine, sports rehabilitation, and clinical psychology specializing in advanced healing techniques. She has 20 years of training and practice in mind-body, self-regulation techniques. Dr. Scott combines her knowledge of science and self-healing in her clinical settings, highlighted by using the left/right brain neuro rebalancing technique for self-healing. She teaches at California Pacific Medical Center, the Institute for Health and Healing, and the University of the Pacific School of Dentistry. She's also a founder, director, and contributing researcher at the Chronic Pain Institute. In her private practice, she teaches Anusara yoga and yoga therapy classes, biofeedback training, and alternative psychotherapy. Her mission is to assist her students in discovering their own greatness and to awaken her students' passion for yoga and all its gifts.

Dedication

This book is dedicated to "The Spirit That Lives Within You."

Authors' Acknowledgments

Joint Acknowledgments: For the photographs in this book, we wish to thank photographer Bonnie Kamin Morrisey for her expertise and her excellent photos; a picture is worth a thousand words. Many thanks as well go to all the models from Sherri's yoga classes who posed for photographs: Linda Prosche, Allan Carr, Marian Jung, Christine Bandettini, Nick Freeman, William Keller, and Justine Rudman (and her baby within). We would also like to thank Paula and Andy Valla for crossing the Iron Man Triathlon finish line in Chapter 16 and for being our yoga-with-weights champions. Thanks as well go to Carol Jones for handling the models' makeup and to Stress Management Center of Marin for its beautiful studio. We would also like to thank Magaña Baptiste for the vintage photos of herself with her husband, Walt Baptiste.

Project Editor Alissa Schwipps steered this book forward, Copy Editor Josh Dials saw to its clarity, and Acquisitions Editor Mikal E. Belicove encouraged us to take the leap of faith; we're grateful to each of them. We also wish to thank Linda Sparrowe, author and teacher, for serving as this book's technical editor. The treats of good coffee and dark chocolate as we worked through the pages of this book along with pets Bodhi, Sage, and Mollie are all in the mix, too.

They say to see clearly, you should stand on the shoulders of a giant. Our giant in this book is Peter Weverka. He's our experienced wordsmith and skilled writer who helped to sculpt and shape the information found on every page of this book. We know of no other way to acknowledge our gratitude and appreciation for his professionalism and guidance in the process of writing this book than to just say, "Thank you!"

Additional Acknowledgments from Sherri: I wish to express my personal gratitude to those who made this work possible. First, thanks to Larry Payne, PhD, author and friend, for recommending me to Wiley Publishing. Larry told me that writing a book takes on a unique story of its own with many wonderful players in the story. I want to thank my "guiding light," author Karen Leland, for her guidance, friendship, and open heart, and Elson Haas, MD, associate and friend, for giving his time and lending his support. Most of all, my love, gratitude, and sincere appreciation go to Megan Scott, PhD, because without her unending inspiration, contributions, and expertise in the science of physiology, yoga, and physical culture, this book wouldn't be what it is today. We've developed new territory and solid groundwork together with the revolutionary yoga-with-weights system.

I believe that the timeless principles and knowledge so relevant and perfect for today — the principles found in this book — stem from those who walked this path before us and pioneered the way. I'd like to thank my parents, Magaña and Walt Baptiste, for all their love and encouragement through the years; they are pioneers and giants in the fields of health and fitness, human potential, and yoga. My love also goes to my sister Devi and my brother Baron. I'm deeply grateful to my husband Michael David Freeman and our children, Vanessa, Nicole, Nicholas, and Connor, for their support and great spirit during the writing of this book. Most of all, my thanks — beyond words — goes to all my students who, by their commitment and presence in class, nudged me to grow and expand. As their teacher, I have the space to speak my authentic voice and be true to who "I AM."

Additional Acknowledgments from Megan: I would like to thank Sherri Baptiste, who shared her knowledge, beauty, and expertise in the elegant creation of this book. Without her blazing the way with her strong passion for yoga and teaching, this book wouldn't have been written. I thank her for all the long hours of work we shared together in her home, for providing treats and yummy coffee, for her patience and willingness to face the challenges that come with writing a book, and for co-creation and friendship at its best.

I would also like to acknowledge with love and gratitude my parents, who have always encouraged and supported me in my life journey and have lived the example for me to follow; my siblings, who have been my greatest cheering section; and my husband, Ben Messana, MD, who provided more technical support, medical expertise, and advisement than one could imagine. Gratitude and appreciation also go to John Friend, my most cherished yoga teacher, who taught me more than any book or degree could ever touch upon; without his guidance and support in my yoga career, I wouldn't be where I am today. I offer love and gratitude to the Anusara yoga community for providing encouragement, support, joy, and laughter, always helping each other along the way; Desiree Rumbaugh, a masterful teacher who has taught me depth and understanding of the principles of alignment and living life with grace; and to my yoga students who have taught me so much — I honor and value each and every one of them.

Publisher's Acknowledgments

We're proud of this book; please send us your comments through our Dummies online registration form located at www.dummies.com/register/.

Some of the people who helped bring this book to market include the following:

Acquisitions, Editorial, and Media Development

Senior Project Editor: Alissa Schwipps

Acquisitions Editors: Michael Belicove, Michael Lewis

Copy Editor: Josh Dials

Editorial Program Assistant: Courtney Allen

Technical Editor: Linda Sparrowe

Senior Editorial Manager: Jennifer Ehrlich

Editorial Assistants: Hanna Scott, Nadine Bell

Cover Photo: © Bonnie Kamin

Cartoons: Rich Tennant (www.the5thwave.com)

Composition Services

Project Coordinator: Jennifer Theriot

Layout and Graphics: Andrea Dahl, Joyce Haughey, Stephanie D. Jumper, Barbara Moore, Barry Offringa, Brent Savage, Ronald Terry

Photographs: Bonnie Kamin, www.bonnie kamin.com

Illustrations: IUSM Office of Visual Media and Kathryn Born, MA

Proofreaders: Laura Albert, Leeann Harney, Jessica Kramer, Aptara

Indexer: Aptara

Special Help: Sarah Faulkner

Publishing and Editorial for Consumer Dummies

Diane Graves Steele, Vice President and Publisher, Consumer Dummies

Joyce Pepple, Acquisitions Director, Consumer Dummies

Kristin A. Cocks, Product Development Director, Consumer Dummies

Michael Spring, Vice President and Publisher, Travel

Kelly Regan, Editorial Director, Travel

Publishing for Technology Dummies

Andy Cummings, Vice President and Publisher, Dummies Technology/General User

Composition Services

Gerry Fahey, Vice President of Production Services

Debbie Stailey, Director of Composition Services

Contents at a Glance

Table of Contents

Introduction

. . . .

Yoga with weights is the newest incarnation in a long line of yoga-based exercise programs. Yoga itself is at least 5,000 years old; yoga exercising — what we know as *yoga postures* — emerged about 600 years ago. Over the centuries, yoga evolved as it traveled to new cultures, and its practitioners have refined it. Yoga is based on universal principles that appeal to its practitioners on every level — mentally, physically and spiritually. It effects deep change. The discipline acquires a new significance for each generation that encounters it.

What's different about yoga with weights? If you haven't guessed already, yoga-with-weights practitioners carry weights in their hands and strap weights to their ankles as they exercise. Weights add another dimension to yoga; they stabilize your body and engage you more deeply into the yoga exercises. All the physical benefits of traditional yoga — muscle toning, balance, and flexibility — come faster because yoga with weights is more intense and dynamic than traditional yoga. Yoga with weights creates a balance of strength and flexibility. You notice an increase in vitality and an overall sense of well-being. Each time you practice leaves you feeling a little bit better, and, cumulatively, the workouts have enormous health benefits.

Like traditional yoga, yoga with weights is a practice of mind, body, breath, and spirit. Within every exercise you have the ability to harness the power of yoga and bring alive these great Eastern teachings in practical ways that will serve you in your daily living. This book represents a golden opportunity to start down the road to good health and well-being.

About This Book

Yoga with weights is a new exercise program. You won't find the exercises we describe in this book anywhere else. We have three goals in writing this book: to clearly explain the benefits of yoga with weights, safely instruct you in the practice, and motivate you to do the workouts.

Between us, we have 65 years of experience with yoga. Sherri, daughter of the American yoga pioneers Walt and Magaña Baptiste, has been associated with yoga since she took her first baby steps or assumed her first lotus position, whichever came first. Sherri followed in her parents' footsteps, founding "Baptiste Power of Yoga," a nationally recognized yoga method. Sherri has been teaching since her teens and hosting yoga classes, workshops, and retreats for 14 years. Megan, a doctor of integrative medicine, has 20 years of training and practice in mind-body self-regulation techniques. She studied in her college years with Walt Baptiste and has extensive training in Anusara yoga, a discipline that specializes in living with grace and mastering the alignment principals. Megan has been teaching yoga therapy classes for ten years.

We called upon our collective experience with yoga, our understanding of how to teach yoga, and our experience with physical culture practices to create the exercises you find in this book. Some of the exercises are modifications of traditional yoga poses (the *asanas*); others are exercises we developed ourselves to complement traditional yoga. All the exercises are rooted in the classic yoga principles that cultivate the quality of the mind as well as the body. We want every exercise to strengthen your body, build your physical stamina, and cultivate your overall health and well-being. We also make every effort to pay attention to your safety and not put you in a position where you could injure yourself. As long as you follow our instructions, pay attention to your breathing, and consciously remain aware of your body and its needs in the course of exercising, you can be confident about doing your yoga-with-weights workout without getting injured.

We divide the exercises into several different workouts. For example, we offer practical exercises to relieve stress, plus stamina-building, total-body, and energy workouts. We also provide instructions so you can create a yoga-with-weights workout tailored to your health needs and goals. All the exercises in this book are illustrated with photos so you know exactly how to move your body in the exercises.

Another great feature of this book is that you don't have to read it from start to finish; you can dip in wherever your curiosity gets the best of you. The table of contents and the index guide you in your quest to find the information and exercises you need. Or, you can do it the old-fashioned way, reading the book from cover to cover. It's up to you.

Conventions Used in This Book

We want you to understand all the instructions in this book, and in that spirit, we adopted a few conventions:

✔ We explain exercises in numbered steps, which are formatted in **bold.** Follow Step 1 first, and then Step 2 . . . just kidding, you know the drill. But we do recommend you read through each exercise before diving in.

✔ Foreign terms, including Sanskrit terms, appear in *italics.* (Sanskrit is considered the language of spirituality and is used in the ancient texts of India, the country where yoga originated.) Don't worry; we follow every italicized term with a clear definition.

✔ All Web addresses appear in `monofont` for easy identification.

That's not too many conventions, is it? You could almost say that this book is unconventional.

Foolish Assumptions

Pardon us, but we made some assumptions about you, the readers of this book. We assumed that

✔ You want to be in good health.

✔ You're looking for a workout that will make you stronger, healthier, more balanced, and more flexible.

✔ You have little or no background in yoga, yoga with weights, or weightlifting.

✔ You want a book that explains yoga with weights in simple terms that you can understand and put to good use easily.

✔ You want a practice for body, mind, and spirit, and you want to dive into a deeper, more meaningful exercise practice.

✔ If you're a senior citizen, you're looking for exercise techniques that will help you be stronger and more limber.

✔ If you're pregnant, you want to exercise during your pregnancy so you can have an easier childbirth and a healthier baby.

✔ If you're in love with a certain sport — running, swimming, or baseball, for example — you want to get better at the sport you love.

✔ If you're a yoga or fitness instructor, you want to know what yoga with weights is all about so you can teach it.

✔ Above all else, you want to feel great and look your best!

How This Book Is Organized

This book is organized into six neat parts. Here's a brief description of what you'll find in this book so you can get the lay of the land and decide where you want to start poking around first.

Part I: Getting Started

Part I describes what yoga with weights is, how the program differs from yoga and weightlifting, and how it can help your body, mind, and spirit. You discover what equipment you need and how to prepare yourself for your first workout. You look into all-important safety issues so you know right away that you'll be safe doing yoga with weights. And we tell you how to manage exercise pain and discomfort and how to set up a place in your home or office for yoga-with-weights workouts.

Part II: Mastering the Basics

Part II explores yoga-with-weights breathing — you discover different breathing techniques and why conscious breathing is so good for your health — and also delves into the mental side of yoga with weights. You find out how to get motivated to exercise and discover different mental-relaxation techniques. After you prepare your mind for your workout, you can move into the warm-up phase; Part II presents your first yoga-with-weights workout: the Balanced Workout, a total-body workout.

Part III: Refining Your Technique

Part III contains — count 'em — five yoga-with-weights workouts, each one designed to improve your health and conditioning in a different way. You find workouts for toning, energizing, strengthening, or restoring your body. You can also do a workout designed to burn your body fat and trim your love handles.

Part IV: Personalizing Your Program

Part IV is for people who want to tailor their yoga-with-weights exercise programs to their own health goals. You find out how to address specific aches and pains in your body with different yoga-with-weights exercises, how to tone and strengthen — that is, target — specific parts of your body with the exercises, and you find some tasty, wholesome advice for improving your diet.

Part V: Addressing Special Situations

We devote Part V to three groups: athletes, women, and seniors. We provide athletes and weekend warriors with yoga-with-weights exercise programs specific to the sports they love most — swimming, running, soccer, and many others. We provide yoga-with-weights exercises for pregnant women and exercises that address women's health issues. Finally, we offer an exercise program for seniors.

Part VI: The Part of Tens

Part VI gives you, in handy list style, advice for staying motivated as you do yoga-with-weights exercises and for charting your progress. We also dispel ten myths about yoga with weights that may have previously prevented you from trying this exercise program.

But wait — there's more! Turn to the appendix at the end of the book to find yoga Web sites, the names of yoga magazines, and other stuff that helps you discover more about yoga and yoga with weights and get the equipment you need.

Icons Used in This Book

To help you get the most out of this book, we've placed icons here and there to steer you to important and helpful information. Here's what the icons mean.

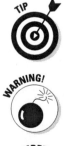

Next to the Tip icon, you find tricks of the trade and helpful hints to make your yoga-with-weights workouts more enjoyable and productive. You also find suggestions about where to look for good equipment and good advice — which helps out your pocketbook and your peace of mind — and how to fit your workouts into your busy schedule.

Where you see the Warning icon, tread softly and carefully. It means we're giving you advice for avoiding injury or doing something that could harm you.

When we provide a juicy fact that bears remembering, we mark it with the Remember icon. When you see this icon, prick up your ears. You'll discover something that you need to remember throughout your adventures in yoga with weights.

We often offer a variation in an exercise — a little twist that makes the exercise either more challenging or a little easier. We mark these variations with the Alternative icon. When you see this icon, you discover a slightly different way to do the exercise. We're here for you in case you want to go the extra mile and, in the case of difficult exercises, when the exercise may be too hard for you.

Where to Go from Here

This book doesn't require a start-to-finish read. However, before you attempt any workouts, we recommend that you check out Chapter 4, which explains yoga-with-weights breathing; you'll be pleasantly surprised to discover how healthy and vital yoga-with-weights breathing makes you feel. We also recommend you check out Chapter 6 about warming up, which all fitness experts agree you should do before exercising.

Other than that, feel free to jump in where the jumping looks best. Think you're ready for your first yoga-with-weights workout? Go to Chapter 7 without passing Go and without collecting $200. Do you need some background information before you undertake yoga with weights? Go to Chapter 1, which introduces this new type of yoga.

Do you have a health goal in mind? Whatever your health goals are, you can find a yoga-with-weights workout in this book to help you on the road to good health. Here are some common health goals and where you should turn in this book to meet those goals:

- **Lose weight.** Who doesn't want to lose a few pounds? See Chapter 11, the Endurance Workout, and Chapter 12, the Belly-Burner Workout.

- **Get stronger.** To increase your body strength, try the exercises in Chapter 10, the Strengthening Workout, and Chapter 11, the Endurance Workout.

- **Reduce stress.** Stress is the silent, slow-acting culprit behind many ailments. To reduce stress, do the exercises in Chapter 7, the Balanced Workout, and Chapter 9, the Restorative Workout.

- **Stay young.** Yoga has a well-deserved reputation for making people look and feel younger. See Chapter 7, the Balanced Workout; Chapter 9, the Restorative Workout; and Chapter 11, the Endurance Workout.

- **Increase stamina.** To give yourself more staying power, see Chapter 11, the Endurance Workout.

- **Sleep better.** If your aim is to get a better night's sleep, check out Chapter 4, breathing techniques; Chapter 7, the Balanced Workout; and Chapter 9, the Restorative Workout.

Chapter 1

Introducing Yoga with Weights

"*W*hat *is* yoga with weights, anyway?" Wonder no more, dear reader. This chapter familiarizes you with this exciting new exercise discipline: what it is, what you can get out of it, and what you need to get started (don't worry, you don't need much).

We believe that everyone can benefit from yoga-with-weights exercises. No matter how flexible you are, how old or young you are, whether you're a paragon of good health or you're just starting down the road to a healthier, happier lifestyle, yoga with weights can help you. We really want to encourage you to take up yoga with weights. We think, no, we *know* you'll love it!

In the Beginning, There Was Yoga . . .

Long before people started working out to dance videos or even doing calisthenics, there was *yoga* — a system of personal development and spiritual practice that began in India at least 5,000 years ago.

You thought yoga was an exercise program, didn't you? If so, you're right. You can get enormous health benefits from yoga exercises, called poses or postures, without going into the spiritual side of yoga.

The eight limbs of yoga

To work toward the goal of self-realization, yoga practitioners study the following eight limbs of yoga and integrate them into their lives:

✔ **Yama:** The code of ethics by which practitioners measure and monitor their behavior. Practitioners refrain from injuring others, lying, stealing, being greedy, and engaging in sensual activities.

✔ **Niyamas:** The observances by which practitioners control their mental energy and develop willpower. The observances are defined as purification, contentment, austerity, sacred study, and attunement to the absolute.

✔ **Asanas:** The poses, or exercises, that constitute the physical aspect of yoga. The exercises help develop the mind-body relationship and build physical strength, flexibility, and balance.

✔ **Pranayama:** The science of Prana (the life force) and its correlation to breathing. By controlling their breathing, practitioners discover how to control their thought processes.

✔ **Pratyahara:** A series of breathing exercises and techniques by which practitioners separate consciousness from sensual perception. The goal is to withdraw the conscious mind from the bondage of the physical body and its instinctual drives.

✔ **Dharana:** A series of breathing techniques and exercises, including mantra, designed to develop endurance through conscious effort and the power of concentration.

✔ **Dhyana:** A series of breathing techniques and exercises designed to help practitioners reach an effortless state of meditation.

✔ **Samadhi:** Advanced breathing exercises and techniques designed to return the individual consciousness to perfect divine unity.

But yoga is more than an exercise program. Yoga means "union" or "to integrate" in *Sanskrit* (the language of yoga). Yoga addresses the whole person, cultivating the mind, the body, and the spiritual potential that you have inside. Classic yoga practitioners seek to be integrated with universal consciousness. They believe that life is a process of purposeful evolution toward a state of self-realization. To achieve this state, they study and live the eight limbs of yoga, or the eightfold path (see the upcoming sidebar for more on this topic). Meditation is one of the vital limbs in this system. The exercise side of yoga emerged about 600 years ago to prepare yoga practitioners for meditation. Sitting for hours in yoga meditation is common, and to make themselves strong enough and supple enough to sit in meditation for long periods of time, yoga practitioners developed yoga poses, or *asanas* in Sanskrit. The poses are only one part of a much larger personal development system that over time becomes a rich lifestyle, but in the Western part of the world, most people think of exercises when they hear the word "yoga."

Yoga schools at a glance

No yoga school is better than another; which one you choose to study is simply a matter of personal preference. More important than any yoga school is the student-teacher relationship.

The differences between schools usually have to do with emphasis. For example, some schools place more emphasis on the alignment of the body, the coordination of breath and movement, holding postures, or the transition from one posture to another.

Roughly speaking, here are the different yoga schools:

✔ **Ananda:** Developed by Swami Kriyananda, a direct disciple of Paramhansa Yogananda. The emphasis is on self-realization.

✔ **Anusara:** As taught by John Friend, this school focuses on flowing with grace and is based on principles and spirals of alignment.

✔ **Ashtanga:** Developed by K. Pattabhi Jois, this yoga gives you a serious athletic workout.

✔ **Baptiste Method of Yoga:** Developed by Magaña and Walt Baptiste, this school is based on Raja yoga; the focus is on mind and meditation.

✔ **Baptiste Power of Yoga:** Developed by Sherri Baptiste, this school brings together flowing postures, breathing techniques, and yoga philosophy.

✔ **Bikram:** Developed by Bikram Choudhury, this school presents a series of 26 static-holding postures practiced in a room heated to 110° Fahrenheit.

✔ **Himalayan Institute:** Developed by Swami Rama from a lineage of sages of the ancient cave monasteries of the Himalayas, the focus is on meditation.

✔ **Integral:** Swami Satchidananda's Integral yoga is a major componenet of Dr. Dean Ornish's groundbreaking work on reversing heart disease.

✔ **Iyengar:** Developed by B.K.S. Iyengar, this school emphasizes attention to detail and the precise alignment of postures.

✔ **Kripalu:** This school puts great emphasis on proper breathing, alignment, and the coordination of breath and movement.

✔ **Kundalini:** Developed by Yogi Bhajan, this school emphasizes classic poses, breathing, the coordination of breath and movement, and meditation.

✔ **Paramahansa Yogananda:** This is the Kriya yoga self-realization fellowship; the emphasis is on the spiritual and on meditation.

✔ **Power Vinyasa Yoga:** Developed by Baron Baptiste, this is a sweat-based, synchronized, dynamic-flow yoga practiced in a room heated to 85–90°F.

✔ **Power Yoga:** This school is based on the Ashtanga repetitive series of postures.

✔ **Sivananda:** This school follows a set structure that includes pranayama, classic asanas, and relaxation.

✔ **Viniyoga:** Developed by Sri T. Krishnamacharya and carried on by his son, T.K.V. Desikachar, this school is a methodology for developing practices for individual conditions and purposes.

✔ **Vivekananda:** This school offers a spiritual brand of yoga.

From a practical point of view, part of the appeal of yoga comes from the stress reduction that occurs while practicing the postures and concentrating on the breathing, which we discuss in detail in Chapter 4. Practice yoga long enough and you'll discover that yoga is a personal journey as well; you notice an overall sense of well-being and peace of mind. Yoga can help you relax, feel more grounded, and experience more joy in your life. For that reason, it benefits not only your mental and physical health, but also the quality of your work and daily life.

In this book, we focus mostly on the physical aspects of yoga with weights. We want you to know that the techniques, exercises, and practices you experience in this system aren't watered down; they're the real deal for body, mind, and spirit. If you're interested in discovering more about the philosophical and spiritual aspects of yoga, we recommend *Yoga For Dummies,* by Georg Feuerstein and Larry Payne (Wiley).

As a spiritual practice and exercise program, yoga continues to evolve, with new schools of yoga and new exercise variations prospering every day. Enter yoga with weights!

. . . And Now There's Yoga with Weights

Yoga with weights is a hybrid of two powerful, time-tested exercise systems: yoga and bodybuilding. Working out with weights is one of the best ways to achieve overall physical fitness, and yoga is renowned as a system of personal development by which you can cultivate peak performance and achieve a higher quality of life. By combining these exercise systems, yoga with weights addresses the needs of your body, but it also goes beyond the physical dimension of your well-being.

Yoga with weights calls for 1-, 3-, or 5-pounds weights on your wrists and/or ankles. The weights stabilize your body and help you achieve a higher level of physical benefit and conditioning. Yoga with weights is a system for the body, mind, and spirit. If you practice diligently, it can be a way of being and living through conscious exercise that leads you to discover your true self.

The addition of the weights makes you feel the effect of the yoga training sooner. The weights train your muscles where to be and where to go. In a beginning yoga practice, several months could go by before you start to "get it." You have to figure out how and where to move different parts of your body. It doesn't take you as long to understand what yoga is about when you practice yoga with weights, because the weights help you move your body into the right positions. The weights force you to engage the right muscles. The added weight also offers a deeper sense of physical grounding, and the weights challenge your balancing skills more intensely than traditional yoga.

The Baptiste family's yoga journey

In his lifetime, Sherri's father, Walt Baptiste, had an interesting yoga journey, one that prefigures yoga with weights. Walt started as a body-builder and later incorporated yoga into his exercise program. Along with his wife (and Sherri's mother) Magaña, he opened the first yoga school in San Francisco in 1955. (Walt and Magaña are pictured here.)

Walt won the "Mr. America" bodybuilding title in 1949. He was the founder and editor of *Body Moderne* magazine, a publication for body-builders devoted to health and fitness. He was always experimenting with ways to improve his bodybuilding techniques, and his experiments eventually led him to breathing and mindfulness techniques. Rather than grunting, groaning, and straining in his bodybuilding workouts, Walt dis-covered how to apply the principals of concen-tration and breath, as practiced today in yoga with weights.

Yoga was considered an extremely exotic prac-tice when Walt and Magaña started teaching classes in the 1950s. Standing on your head,

contemplation, meditation, and contorting your-self seemed too foreign and too strange. For fear of being embarrassed, some of the stu-dents who came to the Baptiste's Yoga Philosophic Health Center in the 1950s asked the couple not to tell their spouses that they were taking these weird "yogurt" classes.

Walt understood that yoga was more than a mere exercise program; he knew that it had the power to transform people's lives and empower individuals in ways that working out simply couldn't. And Walt was right. Now you can see yoga studios and people walking along with rolled-up yoga mats in every major American city. By some estimates, 20 million Americans are taking the yoga journey. Three-quarters of all health clubs offer yoga classes. The yoga-client list includes professional athletes, celebrities, and health professionals. The cur-rent yoga boom is no surprise; its popularity and staying power are testaments to its value as an exercise program that addresses the body, mind, and soul.

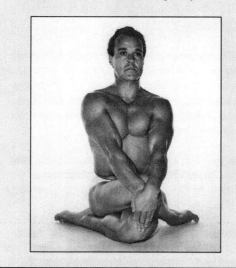

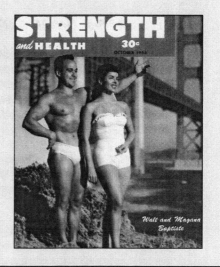

Walt and Magaña Baptiste

Weighing the Benefits of Yoga with Weights

Before you take the plunge and give yoga with weights a try, you may be interested in knowing what the many health benefits of yoga with weights are. Here's a catalog of health benefits you may experience if you devote yourself to yoga with weights.

Making you stronger

Yoga makes you stronger and tones your muscles, but by adding the weights, you give additional boost to the muscle strengthening and toning powers of yoga.

When you stress a muscle with exercise or a repeated activity, the muscle increases in strength and diameter as the muscle fiber expands. In other words, the muscle is toned. The weight-bearing aspect of yoga with weights improves the oxygenation of muscles, which promotes the muscles' growth and repair. The stretching improves the flexibility and health of muscles and tendons. Yoga with weights also reduces the risk of muscle tears and strains because weightlifting, when properly done, integrates the muscles closer to the bones.

Building your core strength

You read a lot about your "core" and "core strength" in this book. When we write about your core, we're referring to the muscles of your trunk and torso that support your spine. These muscles are the major players in balancing and coordination. The core muscles also support your shoulders and hips. Most people don't know it, but the abdominal muscles, which are also core muscles, are very important for supporting your spine.

Unless your core muscles are strong, you can't develop the muscles of your arms and legs to their fullest potential, in much the same way that tree branches can't grow big unless the trunk of the tree is strong enough to support the branches.

Your core muscles are responsible for good posture. They keep your back straight and your shoulders square, and they keep you from slouching. Your core muscles also support and protect your internal organs. For example, if the muscles around your back and abdomen aren't strong, sitting up straight for long periods of time is hard, because the muscles of your back and abdomen take some of the weight-bearing stress off the smaller muscles in your head, neck, and even your shoulders. Without strong core muscles, you're more susceptible to back problems.

When most people think of getting stronger, they imagine being able to lift heavier weights or run faster. But before you can accomplish such feats, you need to develop the core muscles of your trunk and torso. Deep strength begins in these core muscles — your power source, the axis around which so many muscles move. Yoga with weights is a superb program for reaching into the center of your body to engage, utilize, and exercise the core muscles that really matter.

Toning your muscles

Yoga-with-weights exercises are designed to work and tone all the muscles of your body. If you think your arms are too flabby, if you want to develop your abdominal muscles, or if you want to strengthen your legs, you can find many yoga-with-weights exercises that target those areas. In traditional yoga, you can tone and refine parts of your body with exercises. The addition of weights makes it possible to really dig into a muscle or muscle group and work it hard. Chapter 15 describes exercises that target different body areas.

Being more beautiful

Beauty is in the eye of the beholder, of course. But beauty is also a matter of confidence, poise, and bearing. We've seen older people with wrinkles and thinning silver hair who don't fit the standard definition of beauty but who are nevertheless very beautiful. These people radiate an inner glow that has ripened during the years. They have a light in their eyes that tells you that they're very much alive to the world around them and living their lives in a way that's full of enthusiasm. They have what's sometimes called inner beauty or an inspired state of being.

It's often said that yoga slows the aging process. What yoga really does is to help maintain and improve your posture and general health through exercising and proper breathing. Yoga with weights helps to increase your vitality and overall well-being so you look and feel younger and more beautiful. It can give you self-confidence and poise, increase your self-awareness, and make the light inside you shine more brightly with each decade.

Addressing your flexibility and range of motion

Yoga is well known for making people more flexible, supple, lithe, and limber. You've probably seen photographs of human pretzels, like the one in Figure 1-1, contorting themselves into different yoga postures. Being flexible is necessary if you want to be comfortable in your body. Think of all the practical advantages of being flexible. You can reach higher, sit more comfortably on the floor, sit at your desk for longer periods of time with greater ease, or stand longer. You have the choice of bending at the waist or squatting when you want to pick up something from the floor.

Soreness, swelling, and pain relate to the loss of body tissue movement. To prevent injury and postural changes, it helps if your joints have a maximum range of motion.

Many people believe that being flexible enough to get into pretzel poses is the primary goal of yoga. Being flexible does show up over time as a natural part of the process, but it's a secondary goal. You can be a good yoga practitioner without being especially flexible. Yoga with weights combines basic master techniques from the yoga tradition with physical culture practices. The goal is to achieve the proper body alignment and breathe correctly in every move and exercise while cultivating an open mind and heart. You want to achieve a balanced and overall strengthening effect, not to be as flexible as a pretzel.

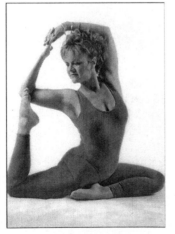

Figure 1-1:
Author
Sherri
Baptiste in a
yoga pretzel
pose.

Indian club, anyone?

If you think yoga with weights is new under the sun, think again. As an exercise discipline, combining yogalike postures with weights is many centuries old, except that the ancient practitioners didn't lift weights as we know them. They lifted heavy wooden clubs called *gadas,* or *Indian clubs*. After the British colonized India, they recognized the value of exercising with Indian clubs, and swinging Indian clubs became an exercise activity in Britain and then in the United States in the late 19th and early 20th centuries. In some respects, yoga with weights is a return to an exercise program that was practiced in India for centuries and was well known to American and British exercise enthusiasts 100 years ago.

Indian clubs are shaped like bowling pins. They range in height from 2 to 2½ feet and weigh between 1 and 7 pounds. If you could time-travel to an American gymnasium in 1910, you'd see an assortment of Indian clubs painted with colorful designs lined up against the wall. The clubs have since become collector's items. Look up "Indian clubs" next time you visit eBay (www.ebay.com), the online auction house. You'll see some beautiful examples.

Physical trainers liked the clubs because they permitted you to build muscle strength while maintaining the range of motion in your arms and shoulders. Exercising with Indian clubs was sometimes called *circular weight training.* In traditional weight training, sometimes called *linear weight training,* you isolate one muscle or one muscle group as you lift. This isolation can make you stiff or muscle-bound after you train for a while. But by swinging Indian clubs, you can build strength while retaining your grace of motion.

Yoga with weights and circular weight training share some common traits. Both work your muscles, and both help your muscles retain their agility, flexibility, and range of motion.

Improving your circulation

Whenever you exercise, you improve your blood circulation. After you stretch or contract a muscle in a yoga-with-weights exercise and the muscle relaxes, it becomes flooded with blood! Flooded with blood may sound like the title of a horror movie, but this blood inundation is good for you because it increases the flow of blood to your muscles, and blood delivers nutrients. Your muscles become stronger and healthier because they receive more nutrients. Stretching also helps renew muscles and muscle fiber.

Creating body awareness

Yoga with weights builds body awareness. You can think of yoga with weights as a dialogue between your mind and body. As you exercise, your brain sends a message to a part of your body telling it to move in a certain direction, and your body sends a signal back to your brain saying that the body part can make the desired motion or can't move any farther. When your brain receives its signal, it sends out another signal asking the part of the body to become more active or relax a little more. This ongoing dialogue amounts to a self-exploration of your body. In a very profound way, it makes you more aware of your body and enables you to extend the physical limits that you thought your body was incapable of reaching.

For the past several years, Sherri has worked with an older man who had polio in his youth. Her experiences with this man have shown her just how beneficial yoga can be to body awareness. He can now bend over, sit up, and walk with more ease, confidence, and coordination. In general, his muscle strength, range of motion, and overall sense of well-being have improved. Through his commitment and practice, yoga has been supportive and helped him rewire some of what we call the nerve highways and pathways that polio had damaged.

Focusing on your balance and coordination

Most of the yoga-with-weights exercises in this book challenge your ability to balance and your coordination. Balancing is discovering how to work muscles in opposition to one another. When you balance on one leg, for example, you flex, or integrate, some muscles, and you relax others. If you flex or relax the wrong muscles, you lose your balance. Yoga with weights helps you understand which muscles to contract or relax in an action, and in so doing it teaches balance and coordination.

Balancing improves your ability to direct your thoughts or stream of concentration. You develop skills of concentration in order to balance. Balancing fires the neurons of your brain. It helps clear the nerve highways and pathways so you can focus better. Recent studies in brain elasticity indicate that exercises that develop coordination and balance stimulate the brain to create new maps and communication pathways, keeping the brain healthy and vital.

Building bone density

Loosely speaking, "bone density" refers to how strong and dense your bones are. To be specific, *bone density* is a measure of how tightly packed the cells and molecules in a bone are. The more tightly packed the tissue is, the higher the bone density, and the healthier the bone. Low bone density increases your risk of fracturing or breaking a bone.

As they age, most people lose bone density, partly because their bodies can't absorb the calcium and minerals they need for strong bones as readily as they once could. Bone density decreases gradually in men and women starting at age 30; in women, the decrease is more pronounced after menopause because estrogen, the ovarian hormone, plays a role in maintaining strong bones.

Weight-bearing exercises such as yoga with weights help bones retain density. When you lift a weight, your muscle pulls against your bones, which makes your bones experience stress. Detecting this stress, your body sends a signal to the cells in your bones that goes something like this: "Please get stronger and denser." Isn't it nice to know that some kinds of stress are actually good for your health?

Finding out the correct way to breathe

"But I know how to breathe," we hear you say. Are you sure about that? Most people don't realize that they aren't breathing correctly. They don't breathe with their abdomens, mid-diaphragm areas, or upper chest areas in a balanced way. Instead, they habitually take short, shallow breaths. When they exercise, some people even hold their breath without realizing it. Most people don't always breathe fully into their lungs, and they miss out on the many wonderful benefits of proper breathing.

We devote an entire chapter to breathing — Chapter 4. Proper breathing can reduce stress and lower your blood pressure. It delivers life-giving oxygen to your body so you have the energy you need. Yoga and yoga with weights are two of a handful of exercise programs that concern themselves with breathing properly. Read Chapter 4 to understand what a deep breath really is.

Squeezing and soaking

Squeeze-and-soak exercises are exercises that massage your internal organs — your liver, stomach, intestines, pancreas, and others. We include many squeeze-and-soak exercises in this book because they help squeeze out the toxins in your internal organs and deliver more blood and oxygen to the organs.

When you bend forward or twist your spine, you squeeze and soak. When you return to a resting position, your organs open up and return to their normal shapes and sizes, and as they do so, they soak up oxygenated blood cells. This oxygenation restores and helps to maintain the organs' health and vitality.

Developing the quality of self-awareness

This book mostly sticks to the physical side of yoga with weights, but that doesn't mean we want to downplay the quality of consciousness and self-awareness that yoga practitioners develop when they commit themselves deeply and intensely to yoga. Yoga consciousness is real. Yoga encourages you to be more aware not only of your body, but also of the world around you.

The discipline helps you stay in the moment so you're more cognizant of sounds, sights, and other sensations. Yoga awakens you. It teaches you to live a life without blinders so you're more keenly in tune with the flow of life — the mysterious force that makes the world pulsate and grow.

We like to compare the yoga practice to the opening of a rose or other flower. The roots, foundation, and stem of the rose — the flower's physical body — must be strong enough to support it. Yoga-with-weights exercises strengthen your body. As the flower awakens, it blossoms and opens its petals to drink in the sunlight. Similarly, the meditation and breathwork that accompany the yoga-with-weights practice open your awareness to the outside world and your own potential to grow. Like the blossoming rose absorbing light from the sun, you commune and connect from within more completely with the world around you.

Evaluating Your Readiness

"Can I really do this?" is a question many people ask themselves everyday. But when they ask this question, they ought to remember that the only thing that gets in their way, most of the time, is themselves. They invent excuses *not* to try a new activity even if the activity is very good for them. Everybody is good at procrastinating. The discussion that follows is for people who can't quite decide whether yoga with weights is for them.

You haven't studied yoga

Should you have studied yoga already in order to study yoga with weights? The short answer is: It isn't necessary. Yoga with weights is user-friendly, meaning it isn't intimidating, and you don't need a background in yoga. The door is always open. Anyone who's interested is welcome.

Yogis sometimes say, "You're as young as your yoga practice." The saying refers to yoga's rejuvenating qualities and to the fact that practicing yoga is akin to being a newborn, in that you discover anew how to move your body when you practice yoga. Like a baby learning to lift his or her head or roll over, yoga students feel their way into new, more liberating body motions and positions as they practice yoga. Yoga is well known for making people look and feel younger. To some degree, yoga slows down the aging process. Bone mass develops, and you feel more vital and energetic.

Of course, if you've already studied yoga, studying yoga with weights is that much easier because the language and the concepts aren't completely new or unfamiliar. For example, you already understand the importance of breathing in exercise. If this book instructs you to breathe deep into your chest and lungs, you know what's what. And if this book tells you to move into the downward-facing dog position, you know exactly what that is. A downward-facing dog? Don't all dogs face downward?

You haven't had weight training (or you lift weights on the regular)

You don't need to have lifted weights before now to study yoga with weights. The weights you use are only 1 to 5 pounds and aren't difficult to get the hang of. If you've never picked up a weight before, rest reassured that holding a pair of hand weights or strapping on a pair of ankle weights doesn't take any expertise whatsoever. The weights help you feel more grounded but don't weigh you down.

We've noticed that the yoga room intimidates people who have lifted weights. Why? Because weightlifters aren't flexible, and they're used to being some of the fittest, best athletes in the gym. Sherri can't count the number of times weight trainers and big-time bodybuilders have told her, "I really want to come to your yoga class." But only a handful of them showed up.

Stepping out of your element and comfort zone is a challenge for everybody, bodybuilders included, but taking that first step is actually much easier than you may think. The real beauty of yoga with weights for people who do lift weights regularly is that it benefits them in new and balanced ways, allowing them to reclaim full range of motion and flexibility while maintaining their strength. This is just what they often need.

One of the biggest attractions of yoga with weights is being able to lift weights and still maintain your flexibility. You get the same muscular tone you get from weight training and work on your flexibility as well. You won't get "bulked up" or muscle-bound, but your muscles will be toned, defined, and strengthened.

You're really out of shape

Out of shape? Who? You? Well, you're not the only one who's out of shape. Life just starts doing its thing with us and pretty soon we fall out of shape. We're sure you've been told before that staying in shape takes consistency and a life-long commitment. All you have to do is put in the effort and you soon reap the rewards.

If you're very out of shape, start slow. Go to Chapter 6 and start with the gentle walking and breathing exercises. Try to observe a daily walking program of 20 to 45 minutes to get the ball rolling. When you build your confidence, go to Chapter 7 and start doing the Balanced Workout. You may also want to check out Chapter 18, which offers low-impact exercises designed for seniors.

Busy moms, CEOs, and other dynamic people we know use this technique to find time to exercise: They schedule the time. Knowing how easy it is *not* to exercise, they enter their yoga classes on their calendars and plan their time around yoga. They make a commitment in writing to show up. The classes are on their calendars and they have to go no matter what. (Chapter 19 provides you with some tips for staying motivated to work out.)

You're stiff as a board

Some people are by nature muscle-bound or tight, and they have a limited range of motion. They can hardly lean forward far enough to tie their shoes.

People with tight muscles tend to be protective and guarded in their movements. They don't have the confidence to move freely. This lack of confidence hinders their movements and makes them even stiffer. Eventually, they may develop bad posture, which can lead to other health problems, including chronic back pain and chronic headaches (see Chapter 14). Bad posture can compress the internal organs, causing poor digestion, high blood pressure, and respiratory ailments.

If you're stiff by nature, yoga with weights can seem like a risky enterprise mentally and emotionally when you begin exercising. But hang in there. Breath by breath, exercise by exercise, you can escape the cage that your body has become, spread your wings, and fly. As Chapter 4 explains, yoga breathing techniques can improve the blood circulation in your body and bring new healthy cells to your muscles. Where flexibility is concerned, success breeds success. One muscle unknotting can cause the one beside it to loosen. Even people who are very stiff by nature can become limber if they stick with yoga with weights and practice it as little as twice a week. Eventually, your muscles will rest back against your bones and stretch out and elongate, and you'll be able to move more comfortably and freely.

You're loose as a goose

Some people are double-jointed. Their tendons and ligaments are more elastic. They can touch their noses to their knees without any distress or bend over backwards to touch the floor. People who are double-jointed, or hyperflexible, run the risk of hyperextending their knees, elbows, and other joints because their ligaments and tendons are too elastic. They're capable of flexing well beyond a joint's normal range. Unless they develop the muscular strength to support their supple joints, these people can injure their joints in the course of doing an exercise.

Hyperflexibility is probably a matter of genetics. You're born with limbs that are too loose, but you can do something about it. Yoga with weights can benefit people who suffer from hyperflexibility because it strengthens supporting muscles. This extra muscle mass makes the joints more stable.

You're pregnant or have a preexisting medical condition

A few medical conditions may preclude you from doing yoga with weights. If you have a heart condition, you're obese, or you're pregnant, think twice before undertaking this form of exercise and proceed with caution. You may have to consult your doctor before doing the exercises.

The cardinal rule of yoga applies especially to people with medical conditions: If something doesn't feel right, if an exercise makes you uncomfortable, or if you feel pain, don't do it. Back away from the exercise and consider whether you're doing it right or whether you should be doing it at all.

Heart conditions

Heart disease is caused by poor diet, lack of exercise, or a genetic predisposition. The most common heart ailment is *coronary artery disease,* which is caused by a clogging or narrowing of the arteries that restricts the supply of oxygen and nutrients to the heart. If the heart muscle is weakened and can't pump blood efficiently, *congestive heart failure* can result. Signs of a heart condition include angina (chest pain or discomfort that occurs when your heart muscle doesn't get enough blood), edema (swelling in the legs), and shortness of breath.

If you have a heart condition such as coronary artery disease, speak to your doctor before you undertake any kind of exercise. All forms of exercise, including yoga with weights, place a burden on your cardiovascular system because exercise increases the flow of blood and stresses the heart muscle. For that reason, you must be especially careful before you undertake an exercise program if you have a heart condition.

The good news for people who are cleared by their doctors to practice yoga with weights is that the discipline offers real rewards to patients with heart disease. Yoga with weights lowers your stress level and gives you the opportunity to exercise at your own pace without overtaxing your cardiovascular system.

Obesity

Being obese doesn't prevent you from doing yoga with weights, although you do have to start slowly. If the Balanced Workout exercises we describe in Chapter 7 are too difficult, start with the chair exercises we present in Chapter 18. You'll discover that after a few workouts, the core muscles in your trunk and torso will become stronger. The weight on your body will be distributed more evenly and you'll be able to move more freely.

Pregnancy

Before you take on yoga with weights or another new exercise program during a pregnancy, seek the advice of a prenatal care physician. Typically, women who have been cleared to exercise can do most of the standing and sitting exercises we describe in this book until the fifth or sixth month of pregnancy. After that period, depending on the woman and how strong she feels, doing exercises that require lying on your back or belly may be too strenuous or difficult.

In our experience, women who practiced yoga before they became pregnant can continue doing many of the standard yoga practices throughout their pregnancies, but women who want to take up the discipline to stay healthy during their pregnancies are better off in prenatal yoga classes. The trainers who oversee these classes know which exercises are suitable for pregnant women; they're attuned to a pregnant woman's health and understand how to guide her through yoga workouts. Chapter 17 has advice for pregnant women who want to study yoga with weights.

What You Need to Get Started

To get started with yoga with weights, you need a little willpower, an open mind, and a sense of adventure; at least those are the only intangibles you need. Taking the first step in any new activity is usually the hardest part. Go ahead and take the first step. You won't regret it.

As for the tangibles, you need some equipment to get going. You need a quiet and comfortable place to exercise, hand weights, and ankle weights. Chapter 2 explains all the equipment in more detail.

Mastering Posture Alignment Techniques

Posture alignment refers to how your muscles are integrated and bones are aligned to support your body for optimal movement during exercise. The aim of good posture alignment is to establish a solid foundation with your body so you can support your limbs, back, and head while you exercise. You want your body to be safe, secure, and able to expand more fully and freely during each exercise.

To avoid injury and to get more out of yoga-with-weights exercises, it pays to practice proper posture alignment. The posture-alignment techniques we present here give you a greater sense of stability and balance not only when you exercise, but also when you stand in lines or sit for long periods of time. The better your posture is, the fewer injuries you're prone to in exercise and in daily life.

In the workout chapters in this book, we often give directions for maintaining a solid foundation. Here are the directions you come across in the exercise descriptions that deal with posture alignment:

- ✓ **Engage your core muscles.** Your core muscles are the muscles in your trunk and torso that are responsible for supporting your spine. When you engage these muscles, it feels as though you're wearing a tight-fitting spandex suit on your body because you have a "hugged-in" feeling. You feel empowered when you move from your core muscles into all the exercises.

- ✓ **Draw your belly in and up and your tailbone down.** As your tailbone drops toward the floor, your legs strengthen, and you press your leg muscles up against the bone where they can support your body. You should feel the muscles hugging the bones as the bones begin lengthening.

- ✓ **Press into all four corners of your feet.** You root downward through the soles of your feet to create depth and stability while you exercise. You should feel equal weight on the front and back of each foot as well as on the sides. Feel the corners of your heel and the ball or pad on the front of your foot — especially the area below your big toe and baby toes — pressing downward. You should also feel the arches of your feet gently lifting up as if energy from the front of your shins is pulling your arches up. The feeling continues through your knees as your thigh muscles gently lift your knees upward.

- ✓ **Stabilize and center your head between your shoulders.** We may ask you to perform this action during standing exercises. Gaze forward with your chin naturally down, not lifted or tilted. Draw your shoulders away from your ears and your shoulder blades down your back. Make sure your chest is comfortable, spread your collarbones wide, and give a slight lift to your breast bone or sternum, lifting naturally. Stand with your hips aligned over your knees and with your knees over your heels.

- ✓ **Spread your fingers wide.** When your hands are on the floor and you're supporting your body with your hands, we ask you to spread your fingers wide so that each finger is active and pressing firmly on the floor to help support your body.

- ✓ **Place your shoulders over your wrists and hands and your hips over your knees.** We give you this instruction when an exercise requires you to be on all fours. When you're in this position, make sure that you distribute your body weight evenly over your wrists, hands, and knees and that you fully engage the core muscles of your trunk.

When you're lifting a hand weight or an ankle weight, always make sure not to hurry. Lift the weight in a slow, controlled fashion. When you go slow, you make your body more stable and capable of supporting the weight, you isolate the muscle you want to work more effectively, and you don't cheat by relying on your momentum to lift the weight.

No matter what yoga-with-weights exercise you're doing, your entire body should be involved. In addition to keeping your core body engaged, before you do an exercise, direct your thoughts to the specific area that's most actively involved in that particular exercise. For example, if you're doing bicep curls, focus on your biceps. By directing your mind to the specific body action, you enhance your body-mind connection and create a more empowered workout. This technique is also excellent for mental conditioning.

Heeding the All-Important Safety Issues

Use common sense when practicing yoga with weights. If something doesn't feel right, don't do it. Work at your own level of ability and never push yourself too far. The following pages present guidelines for making sure you practice yoga with weights safely. These guidelines can help you determine what's safe, but practically speaking, it's up to you to draw your own guidelines. Yoga with weights is a voyage of self-discovery. After you practice the discipline long enough, you understand what your breathing, discomfort level, and pain level mean. The object of the exercises is to come to the edge without stepping off the cliff — to push yourself without pushing too far. As long as you stay in the moment and register the sensations in your body very carefully, your breathing, discomfort level, and pain level can tell you where the edge is and show you how to get the most from the exercises.

Listen to your breathing

Rapid breathing, short and shallow breathing, holding your breath, and gasping are signs of distress. If you can't take slow, deep, rhythmic breaths as you exercise, you're overexerting and subjecting yourself to injury. Ease away from what you're doing just enough to regain control over your breathing, and then continue with the exercise.

Yoga-with-weights exercising isn't about coming to the edge and falling off; it's about riding the crest of the wave in all its glory and enjoying the ride in the process. For more information on proper breathing techniques, see Chapter 4.

Be aware of your discomfort level

In yoga with weights, you make a distinction between comfortable discomfort and uncomfortable discomfort. Feeling comfortable discomfort, such as the uneasiness that accompanies breaking new ground in yoga with weights (or any other exercise technique), is fine. If you feel uncomfortable discomfort, however, you're straining yourself. Abandon the exercise you're doing and ask yourself whether you're doing the exercise correctly or pushing yourself too far.

Can children study yoga with weights?

Some parents are concerned that working with weights can stunt children's growth. This concern isn't unwarranted. Lifting heavy weights without using the proper technique can put too much stress on the growth plate — the area of growing tissue at the end of long bones — and retard bone growth. If your children lift weights, make sure that they use the proper technique and start with light weights before moving on to heavy ones.

Bone growth, however, isn't an issue for children who practice yoga with weights. The 1-, 3-, or 5-pound weights are light and shouldn't damage growth plates in a child's bones. But if in doubt, have children do the exercises without weights or use the lightest weights. Give your children a lightweight wooden dowel or other item to help them figure out the exercises. They can still get a wonderful workout without the weights.

Getting children to practice yoga with weights isn't easy. Staying in one place is hard for them, and focusing on breathing isn't something they're accustomed to. Children prefer fast-moving aerobic exercises to quiet, contemplative, inward-looking exercise techniques. Still, we encourage parents to get their children to try yoga with weights by making it fun, playful, and not too serious. Besides the physical benefits of discovering balance and coordination, children discover how to direct their minds and concentrate better. Kids who practice yoga with weights often do better in school. They know how to focus and concentrate on the activity before them.

To encourage children to practice yoga with weights, keep the workouts to 30 minutes or less. Try to make a game of the exercises. Children always exercise better in groups, and if you can get a group of kids to study yoga with weights, so much the better. We hope that the addition of weights to the yoga practice will make yoga more attractive to children.

The following photograph shows a young Sherri Baptiste working out with her parents, Walter and Magaña. As you can see, Sherri is lifting a weight. Weightlifting didn't stunt her growth, and she's now considerably taller than she is in this photograph.

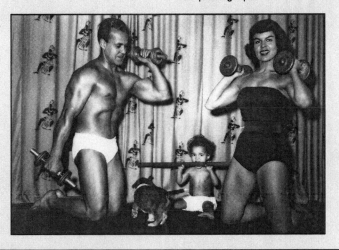

Be aware of any pain you feel

As with other exercise techniques, you sometimes feel pain when you do yoga-with-weights exercises. Pay careful attention to any pain or discomfort you feel. Listen to it. Focus on the part of your body where the pain is located. Burning or stinging pain signals you to be careful, but not necessarily to back away from what you're doing. Sometimes you can control this kind of pain by breathing. Quivering or sharp pain means you've gone too far. You're pulling muscle off the bone and subjecting yourself to injury.

Practice at a slow but steady pace

When you're exercising, switching to automatic pilot and going through the motions is easy. When that happens, you increase your chances of injuring yourself, because you're not focusing on your body. Listen to your body and focus on what you feel as you exercise. This, along with conscious breathing and a steady exercise pace, helps prevent injuries. We carefully designed every exercise in this book to give you a workout but spare you the risk of injury. Timing and proper breathing are the keys to the depth and success of each workout and practice. Try not to speed up to get your workout over with quickly. By the same token, don't go so slow that you lose your pacing and rhythm and make the workout boring.

Chapter 2

Gearing Up

*Y*oga with weights doesn't require as much gear as a trip across Antarctica, where the slippery surfaces make for some tough yoga conditions, but you do need a few items. The bare necessities are hand and ankle weights, but we also recommend that you have a yoga mat, the right clothes, good shoes (for warming up), and water for staying hydrated as you work out. The good news for you? These items don't cost a bundle.

Read on for more information about the gear and equipment you need — some of it shown in Figure 2-1 — for a yoga-with-weights workout.

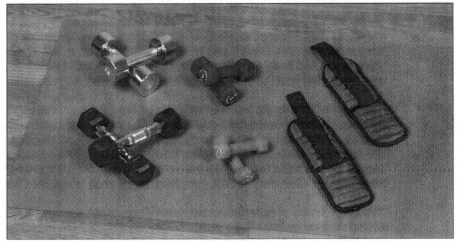

Figure 2-1:
Some of the accoutrements you need for a yoga-with-weights workout.

Weighing Your Hand- and Ankle-Weight Options

You need two kinds of weights if you want to incorporate weight resistance into your yoga workouts: hand weights to hold and ankle weights to strap to your ankles. Most sporting goods and athletic stores carry these weights, and you may be able to find them in the sporting goods sections of department stores. (The appendix lists online stores where you can purchase yoga-with-weights supplies.)

The following sections explain everything you need to know about choosing and using weights, including what size weights you need, the ins and outs of shopping for weights, and a handful of weight accessories that may be useful to you.

Investing in weights of different sizes

We recommend having three sizes of hand and ankle weights at your disposal for your yoga-with weights workouts: a pair of 1-pound weights, a pair of 3-pound weights, and a pair of 5-pound weights.

Always start with the lightest hand or ankle weights and work your way up. This allows you to start from your comfort zone and work your way into the weight that gives you the most fulfilling workout. If you start with the heaviest weight, you run the risk or straining yourself and pulling a muscle.

You may wonder why we don't instruct you to lift weights heavier than 5 pounds. Especially if you're a jock who's been pumping iron in the gym for years, isn't 5 pounds kind of light? You'll discover when you start doing the exercises that 5-pound weights — in addition to the yoga poses — give you a very solid workout. Even if you're an expert weightlifter, the combination of yoga poses and hand weights will test your strength and balancing abilities in new ways that make you sweat and really feel it deep in your muscles.

The yoga-with-weights workout refines and lengthens muscles; it isn't intended to build the bulky body of a Charles Atlas. Yoga with weights creates a leaner, longer, stronger body. The 1-, 3-, or 5-pound weights you use in the exercises stretch your muscles, release tension in your muscles, and engage the muscles in the deep core of your body that you use for balance and stability. (For more on the core muscles of your body, see Chapter 1.)

Not many forms of exercise engage your deep-core balancing muscles. The added resistance from the weights forces your deep-core muscles to spring into action. Lifting weights heavier than 5 pounds may make you too top- or bottom-heavy and upset the balance and distribution of your body weight.

You would no longer focus on balancing or engaging your core muscles; you would exercise your arms or legs in traditional weightlifting fashion.

In the exercise descriptions in this book, we don't tell you which of the three weights to use. The amount of resistance you want is up to you. Experiment with the different weights, and choose the size that gives you the best workout.

Knowing which size weight to use

How do you know which size weight (1-, 3-, or 5-pound) to use in a particular exercise? The size is ultimately up to you, but if you find yourself straining as you do an exercise, consider using a lighter weight.

Here are some telltale signs that you should switch to a lighter weight:

- **Grunting.** Emitting a grunt, a grumble, or a groan in the middle of an exercise means you're straining too much.

- **Holding your breath.** We instruct you when to inhale and exhale when necessary, and we always instruct you to breathe slowly and consciously. If you start holding your breath, it's a sure sign that you're straining to do the exercise.

- **Shaking or cramping muscles.** If your arm, for example, starts shaking or cramping in the middle of an exercise, you're working a particular muscle in your arm too hard. The object of yoga with weights is to engage many muscles at once, not a particular muscle or muscle group.

- **Tiring quickly.** This tells you that you're overambitious where the heaviness of the weights is concerned.

- **Throwing your body.** If you find yourself lunging or throwing your body to lift a weight, you're relying on your momentum to lift rather than your muscles. You've lost your core stability.

Knowing if the weights you're lifting are too light is easy. If you're not working hard enough, switch from 1 to 3 pounds or from 3 to 5 pounds.

Don't be afraid to experiment. Keep different size weights at your side and test the different weights until you find the pair that engages you the best in an exercise. You may find yourself using different weights for different exercises. The surest way to know whether your choice of weights is the right one is to see how you feel after a workout. If your body feels weak and shaky, you need lighter weights; likewise, if you're too sore the next day, you need lighter weights. If you finish a workout with the feeling of "comfortable discomfort" — a feeling that you've met the challenge and given yourself a good workout — you know that your choice in weights was the right one.

Most people exercise with 1- and 3-pound weights. Especially with the ankle weights, 5 pounds can seem like 5 tons when you're in the middle of a workout.

However, we don't want to discourage you from using these weights, especially if you're tall or big.

Shopping for hand and ankle weights

You have many options when shopping for hand and ankle weights. Following are some alternatives and suggestions we provide for your shopping spree.

Hand weights

Sometimes hand weights are sold in sets, and you may be able to find a 1-, 3-, and 5-pound combination. Hand weights are often priced by the pound, with 1 pound costing about $1.50. A 3-pound hand weight, for example, should cost about $4.50.

Recently, a new kind of glove-style hand weight has appeared on store shelves. You can slip your hand into these weights, which gives you an advantage because you don't have to grasp the weight as you lift it, and you can stretch out the fingers of your hand as you move through each exercise. Glove-style weights give you the opportunity to stretch and lift at the same time, and you may even get more of a stretch without the hindrance of carrying or gripping the weights and balancing at the same time. (Look in the appendix for advice for finding glove-style weights on the Internet.)

You have other options if you want to stick to hand-held weights. Weightlifters are accustomed to wearing special fingerless grip gloves that secure the weights in their hands and prevent calluses. If you like grip gloves, by all means use them in yoga-with-weights exercises; just be sure to air out the gloves when you're finished using them.

Never drop a hand weight. When you're done with it, place it carefully on the floor where no one can step on it. And keep weights away from children. You can buy special weight racks for storing weights on the cheap.

Ankle weights

We recommend keeping 1-, 3- and 5-pound ankle weights on hand as you perform the exercises in this book. At most, wear 5-pound ankle weights when you do an exercise. The weights should range in price from $15 to $25 a pair.

Changing ankle weights is considerably more trouble than changing hand weights, so you may want to find ankle weights that strap on and off with ease. Ankle weights with Velcro closures are the easiest to get on and off. You can also try to find ankle weights that come with little pockets for inserting metal slugs of different sizes (see the appendix for information about buying these ankle weights). These pocket-pouch ankle weights make it easy to change weight sizes because you don't have to unstrap the weights and put on a different pair.

Dumbbell timeline

People have been lifting weights, or dumbbells, for several centuries. The first dumbbells weren't made for exercise, but for ringing cathedral bells. These bells were quite large and heavy, and some required several men to operate. To develop their skills, bell-ringers practiced with a dumbbell, a weight as heavy as a cathedral bell suspended from a rope. Because this false bell made no sound, it was called a "dumbbell."

Later, the word dumbbell was applied to weights that people used for exercise. The first recorded use of the word dumbbell in weightlifting occurred in 1711, when the Englishman Joseph Addison wrote in *The Spectator:* "For my own part, when I am in Town, I exercise myself an Hour every Morning upon a dumb Bell that is placed in a Corner of my Room, and pleases me the more because it does every thing I require of it in the most profound Silence. My Landlady and her Daughters are so well acquainted with my Hours of Exercise, that they never come into my Room to disturb me whilst I am ringing." Addison was making a pun. His exercise apparatus was called a dumbbell, and when he used it for exercise, his landlady and her daughter (the belles with whom he lived) were silent (they were dumb).

Settling on the Right Yoga Mat

You need a solid, supporting surface to exercise on, and for that reason, we recommend that you use a yoga mat for your safety. Mats give you padding, comfort, and protection, especially for your knees and spine. However, it isn't necessary to have a yoga mat when you do yoga-with-weights exercises. You can exercise on a solid, non-slippery, close-weave type of carpet or clean, dry floor.

If you're taking a yoga-with-weights class in a gym, we recommend bringing your own mat for hygiene purposes. Most gyms offer yoga mats, but they can get very sweaty. Rolling around in your own sweat is much more agreeable and hygienic than rolling around in a stranger's sweat. (The "Washing your yoga mat" sidebar provides instructions for cleaning a yoga mat.)

When you shop for a yoga mat, look for one that stretches a little and gives you good support. Like Goldilocks's porridge, the mat shouldn't be too thick or too thin. Mats range from a fraction of an inch to an inch deep, but depth isn't the real issue — cushioning is. The idea is to get some relief from the hard floor, and although comfort is fine, a spongy mat can be a nuisance because it doesn't give you a solid base to work on. For your purposes, a quarter- to half-inch-thick mat is best because it offers comfort and stability; if you're uncomfortable sitting on the floor or on your knees, get a mat that's on the thick side. Also, the mat should be as long as you are tall plus about 6 inches; in other words, if you're 5'6", find a 6-foot yoga mat.

Washing your yoga mat

You need to wash your yoga mat from time to time. You'll know when it needs washing because your nose will tell you as much. You can buy special soap for washing yoga mats at natural food stores and yoga studios. You can also buy it on the Internet (the appendix lists companies that sell yoga products). Be on the lookout for soaps that make your mat sticky or slippery; we've had good luck with the "Yoga Mat Spray Wash" made by Vermont Soap Works.

To wash your mat, fill the bathtub halfway with water, add a few drops of cleaner (as recommended), swirl the water around to distribute the cleaner, and submerge your mat for a minute. Then apply a sponge or washcloth to each side of the mat. Next, drain the water from the tub and rinse your mat thoroughly with fresh water. Air-dry the mat, but not in direct sunlight; never put a yoga mat in the dryer because it loses its shape. Mats usually take 24 hours to dry thoroughly. Make sure your mat is completely — and we mean completely — dry before rolling it up; otherwise, it will mildew and acquire a terrible smell.

Don't select a foam mat; they're too thick and too short for yoga-with-weights exercises. Foam mats are made for aerobic exercising.

In the yoga community, some ecology-minded practitioners object to using synthetic materials. You can now buy natural rubber mats and mats made from hemp. These mats are considered more "earth friendly." Look for a dense, sturdy mat without a slippery surface (see the appendix in this book for information about obtaining these mats).

Due to the popularity of yoga, every Tom, Dick, and Harriet has gotten into the yoga-mat business, and some manufacturers don't really know what they're doing. People in our yoga classes often complain about the yoga mats they've purchased because the mats wear down quickly, slide across the floor during exercises, and get slippery from sweat. We recommend mats made by Airex, Tapas, and Prana; you can buy these mats at sporting goods stores, and the appendix explains where you can find them on the Internet.

Assembling Your Workout Ensemble

What you wear for a yoga-with-weights workout doesn't especially matter as long as your outer clothes are loose, comfortable, and easy to breathe in. Don't wear shirts and pants that restrict your movements in any way or drag on the floor, and never wear a belt; the waistband of your pants must be loose so your breathing isn't constricted or confined. For the sake of comfort, wear clothes with natural and breathable fibers. You can find these clothes in many sporting goods stores, outdoor outfitters, and yoga retail stores, as well as on the Internet (see the appendix).

For undergarments, women should wear an athletic or Spandex bra that lifts their breasts and presses them into their bodies. For top-heavy women, this is important for balancing as well as for comfort.

Men should wear (and how do we put this delicately?) tight-fitting — but not too tight-fitting — underwear from which no items may escape and see the light of day. We occasionally get horror-story complaints in our yoga classes from students who have witnessed other students violating this important underwear rule.

Spandex running shorts are excellent for yoga with weights. They support your muscles and keep them warm, and they permit you to move without restriction. Prana and other yoga-product manufacturers offer clothing lines designed especially for yoga practitioners. The appendix in this book shows you how to find yoga clothes on the Internet.

Shopping for Shoes

You don't need shoes for a yoga-with-weights workout because balancing starts with your feet, and when your feet are bare, your muscles work more actively to help you balance. So, why do we discuss shoes in this chapter? Because in Chapter 6, we assert that taking a short walk is a necessary warm-up exercise before working out, and assuming you want to walk outdoors, you need good shoes. Here's some advice for getting the right pair of walking shoes:

- ✔ Choose shoes with arch supports that are designed for exercising.

- ✔ Buy a new pair of shoes when your soles start to wear down. Walking and running in worn-out shoes can cause your feet and ankles to collapse, which can strain muscles and tendons in your feet and calves. Worn-out shoes can also cause problems in your lower back, upper back, and shoulders. If you walk and run daily, you probably need a new pair of shoes every six months.

- ✔ Make sure you have enough room inside your shoes for socks and for swelling. Your feet swell when you exercise.

How the heels of your shoes wear down can tell you a lot about your body alignment. If the slope of your shoe heel shows more wear on the outside of the heel, your outer pelvis muscles are weak. If the slope shows more wear on the inside of the heel, your inner-thigh muscles are weak. Any slope in the heels of your shoes means that you're straining your ankles.

Keeping Water on Hand to Stay Hydrated

All exercisers must pay attention to fluid intake, because as you lose water when you exercise, you run the risk of being dehydrated. Some yoga exercises squeeze and soak your kidneys, which releases toxins in your body. You need to drink water to help flush out those toxins. We recommend having water on hand whenever you do yoga-with-weights exercises.

The U.S. government recommends drinking eight glasses of water a day, but how much you need to drink depends on how active you are. People's bodies and levels of activity are different. If you sit at a desk all day, you don't need to drink eight glasses. However, if you're exercising and running about, and especially if you're sweating, you need more than eight glasses. You have to pay attention to the water you drink and how you feel.

You can tell when you're dehydrated by listening to your body:

- You get a dry throat.
- Your lips start sticking together.
- You get a faint headache.
- Your urine is a dark color.

Many people make the mistake of drinking a lot of water right before they exercise. What they don't know is that the water they drink right before a workout or during a workout doesn't hydrate their bodies. The water you drink three to four hours before your workout quenches your body's thirst. Plan ahead and drink plenty of water before you exercise, especially if you work out in a hot room or gym where you sweat profusely. Keep a bottle of water at your side during your workout in case you need to take a sip, because you need to continue replacing the sweat you lose. After your workout, replenish the fluid you lost with a nice glass of fresh water.

If you soak your shirt during a workout, drink more water. Coffee, tea, and soda are dehydrating. For every cup of coffee, tea, or soda you drink during the day, drink an extra 8 ounces of water.

Get a 1.5-liter or 1-quart container of quality drinking water and sip from it throughout the day. Drinking slowly over the course of the day makes for better hydration and absorption of water by your body. Guzzling, on the other hand, doesn't give your body enough time to absorb the water. By carrying a water bottle with you, you can tell at a glance exactly how much water you've consumed, and you know whether you're staying properly hydrated.

If you use plastic bottles to carry your water, look for the kind that don't decompose as readily, because plastic leaches into the water and can be harmful. Stores such as REI (www.rei.com) carry high-quality plastic containers.

Chapter 3

Preparing for Your First Workout

Congratulations on your decision to take the plunge and try out yoga with weights. This chapter ushers you to the next phase of your journey — from your decision to start the workout to your preparations for the workout. We advise you on how to find the time to exercise and make a place in your home for working out. We describe why exercising in front of a mirror is so helpful, and we look into whether heating the room as you exercise is worthwhile. Finally, we examine the pros and cons of listening to music when you exercise, how to choose a class and an instructor if you want to venture out of your home, and the importance of yoga etiquette.

Finding the Time to Exercise

And the number one reason most people give for not exercising is . . . "I can't find the time." Between work, family obligations, and necessary activities such as eating and sleeping, people don't get around to exercising. They just can't find the time, although the fact that they haven't exercised eats away at them all day long.

However, yoga with weights is easier on your schedule than you may think and well worth the sacrifice of your time. One workout will inspire you to do the next because the workouts feel good and you get so much in return for the amount of time you put in. The yoga-with-weights workout has many benefits and advantages over other exercise programs; we look at these advantages here and answer the question, "Why should I sacrifice my time for yoga with weights?"

Some people use lists to help them make the commitment to exercising. When you wake up in the morning, write down the tasks you want to complete during the day, and check off activities on the list as you complete them. This way, you can direct your attention to the task at hand instead of wasting energy and time remembering everything that you have to get done. Include a yoga-with-weights workout on your list to help you prioritize your activities and make room for a workout. You can fit your workout in your schedule, even if it means rearranging your other tasks. (See Chapter 19 for some more motivation to amp up your workout schedule.)

Because minimal space (and equipment) is required

One of the advantages yoga with weights has over other exercise programs is that you can do it anywhere — well, anywhere you can fit a yoga mat. Here are some tips for people who work in offices and for parents at home:

- Close your office door at lunchtime, turn down the lights so it looks like nobody's home, and do the exercises right there.

  Keep a set of hand and ankle weights in your office for occasions when you can exercise.

- If you work in a cubicle and don't have the floor space to exercise, book a conference room for 20 minutes or find a spot outside.

  If you notice your coworkers silently wishing they could exercise along with you, ask them to join in.

- Moms and dads on the go should try to exercise when their children are taking naps or when they're at school. You can also try to find a babysitter for an hour or two.

  Don't feel like you're being selfish by finding time to exercise. By taking good care of yourself, by building more lean muscle mass, and by building the strength and stamina to take care of you and your baby or you and your kids and family, you'll discover peace of mind and newfound energy resources.

Because it's a quick workout

Unlike a running and weightlifting session or a trip to the gym, a yoga-with-weights workout takes only a tiny bit of your day. The timesaving factor shows up in many places:

✔ You get a full-body workout in the same time it would take to work out only one body part in the gym.

✔ You don't get as sweaty and tired, which means you can perhaps skip a shower if you do the exercises at work.

✔ You can work out just about anywhere; you don't have to take the time to travel to and from a gym or yoga studio.

✔ You can practice your breathing and relaxation techniques during your coffee breaks or while you're stuck in traffic.

If cutting a full 20-to-30 minute slot out of your day to exercise is still too problematic or requires you to juggle too many appointments, you can divide the 20-to-30 minute workout into halves or thirds. For example, do the first four exercises in a workout in the morning and the second four exercises in the afternoon. Try keeping this book on your desk. When you come to a lull in your day — you know, one of those sluggish moments when you've finished one task and can't decide which of the numerous other tasks needs your attention — open this book and do a single exercise. If you're a mom or dad at home with the children, sneak off for a minute or two throughout the day and do one exercise. Your mind will feel clearer, and by the end of the day, you'll have completed an entire workout.

Because it replaces snacking

Many people can find time to snack, but they can't seem to set aside time to exercise. Why is that? A yoga-with-weights workout can take as little as 20 minutes, or about twice the 10 minutes you devote to snacking. Why not forego the snack (or just a couple snacking sessions) and do the exercises instead? You can use the time in the mid-afternoon that you usually devote to snacking for exercising, which gives you a bunch of different benefits:

✔ You may get a better energy boost from exercising than you experience from heavy snacking.

Exercising speeds up your metabolism and makes your body more efficient at processing calories and fat, which can help you lose weight and feel more energetic. Your heart beats faster, and your body functions more efficiently.

✔ You spare yourself the guilt and remorse of not exercising and feel happy that you took the time.

✔ You don't add to your daily calorie intake.

✔ You lose excess weight and help to keep your body healthy.

You may also consider skipping a big lunch now and then in favor of a yoga-with-weights workout. Again, you get the energy benefits of eating a light lunch without the excess calories. Or, instead of skipping lunch altogether, have a light and easy-to-digest snack — an energy bar or protein drink, for example — and then work out. Snack with healthy foods when you feel like it. Explore and experiment with your bodily needs to find out which foods work best for you. Getting to know yourself better is part of the fun.

Everyone's metabolism is different, and everyone has a best time for exercising. Yoga with weights requires you to stretch, and some people are too stiff in the morning to stretch. Some people prefer not to exercise at night because it speeds up their metabolism and gives them energy boosts, which makes it hard for them to fall asleep. Most people use trial and error to discover the best times for them to exercise during the day. Listen to your body to understand how exercise affects your daily energy cycles, and discover the best time of day for you to exercise. When you discover that time and decide how often to work out, build a regular exercise schedule for doing yoga-with-weights exercises, and stick to your schedule.

Creating Your Workout Sanctuary at Home

If you intend to do your yoga-with-weights workouts at home, more power to you (see the section "Working Out in a Group Setting" later in this chapter if you want to work out with others). You can carve out a personalized, private place to work out, you can exercise in front of a mirror, and you can adjust the room temperature and other settings to your specifications. We discuss these topics in the pages that follow.

Setting aside some space

Creating a workout space for yoga with weights is easy enough, because you don't need very much space. If you have enough room to fit a yoga mat, you have plenty of space. Section off a corner of a room, a place on the deck, a few square feet in the backyard, or a few square feet on the roof, provided the roof of your house isn't slanted. Or you can keep it simple and create a special, sacred workout place in your home for exercising.

We believe strongly in the benefits of exercising outside if you can manage it. As long as you don't expose yourself to winds or unkind breezes, direct sunlight, or voyeuristic neighbors, the great outdoors is one of the best places for a yoga-with-weights workout. The fresh air adds to the benefits you get from yoga breathing, and you feel more free-spirited and thankful to be alive when you're in nature.

Yoga with weights is different from most exercise programs because it challenges your powers of concentration. In fact, some exercises test and develop your ability to focus more than they do your physical strength. Therefore, you should choose a place to exercise where distractions won't bother you. Not everyone can swing this, of course, but if you're fortunate enough to have a large house or a fenced-in backyard, see if you can devote an area to yoga-with-weights exercises. By establishing a place away from the rigors and demands of your daily life, you'll find it easier to concentrate on your exercises, deep breathing, and meditation. This special room or backyard space can be a source of resilience during difficult and demanding periods.

Keep your yoga mat, weights, and this book in your designated workout area (if your area is inside) so you can start exercising as soon as you set foot in it. You can keep this space simple or decorate it with fitness, yoga, meditation, or spa-style decor. Simple, bare, or elaborate — it's up to you. As soon as you set foot in your area, you should know you're there for one purpose — to work on yoga with weights. Knowing this helps you get into the exercise mindset. Think of your exercise space as a magic land or sanctuary where your health is the utmost concern. As soon as you step into the sanctuary, the exercises begin and nothing else concerns you.

Exercising in front of a mirror

If you have the room to hang a mirror in your exercise area, do so. Exercising in front of a mirror gives you the opportunity to make like a yoga-with-weights instructor and observe your workout so you know when you're making mistakes or doing exercises incorrectly. Apart from showing how beautiful or handsome you are, the mirror shows you when your body is aligned correctly during an exercise. Having the correct alignment is essential in yoga with weights, because the exercises rely on your balance to work different muscle groups and tax the core muscles in your trunk and torso.

Pay attention to whether your body is in proper alignment with the following tips in mind:

- **Posture:** If you stand during an exercise, stand up straight and look straight ahead. Traditional yoga teaches that body energy moves through the spine. Make sure your spine is erect so your body is energized and open.

- **Shoulders:** Don't shrug your shoulders; keep your breast bone gently lifted and your collarbones wide with your shoulders firmly on your back. Don't slouch or cave in. Except for the occasional exercise when we ask you to roll your shoulders forward, you should stay gently lifted in the chest and breathe evenly into your body.

Most people have one shoulder that's higher than the other. Correct this imbalance when you see it in the mirror by consciously breathing into your imbalanced side, as if you're inflating it. This gently unlocks your body and improves your posture.

✔ **Legs:** In exercises in which we ask you to move one foot forward and the other foot back, make sure your legs are balanced and your body weight is equally distributed between both legs. Is one foot too far forward or too far back? You can tell with a glance in the mirror.

✔ **Knees:** In squatlike poses where we ask you to bend your knees and sit in an imaginary chair, some people hardly bend their knees. Don't be afraid to bend them — the movement is good for you. If you have stiff knees, always warm up first (see Chapter 6) and focus on the balls of your feet being on the floor when you bend your knees — this gives you a solid base. Never force or lock your kneecaps back; using your thigh muscles above your knees, gently lift your knees upward and into your thigh bones to strengthen the knee area for greater support.

✔ **Feet:** In most standing exercises, your feet are parallel to one another. Don't turn your feet out. When we ask you to place your feet below your hips or place them "hips' width apart," look to see if your feet are directly below your hips and if your stance isn't wider than your hips.

The only drawback of doing the exercises in front of the mirror is that you may miss the from-the-inside-out experience of yoga. Recognizing and feeling each breath, moment, and exercise from the inside out is what makes yoga with weights an empowering practice. If you gaze in the mirror and look at yourself only from the outside in, you miss an aspect of the exercises and never discover what yoga is really about.

In our classes, we occasionally notice students gazing with puppy love at their reflections in the mirror, and that's okay. Admiring yourself is allowed. Why not? It sometimes happens that someone who feels self-conscious and thinks he or she isn't beautiful discovers otherwise in the mirror. As long as you do the exercises and complete the workout, you're allowed to admire yourself. So strike that pose and then get over it so you can dive deep within yourself for the real rewards.

Use this book as a tool. Compare the exercise photos you see in this book to your reflection in the mirror to find out whether you're striking the right poses as you exercise.

Turning up (or turning down) the heat

Some yoga instructors and yoga schools believe in heating the exercise room. The idea is for the excess heat to warm and loosen your muscles, making them easier to stretch. People turn up the thermostats in exercise rooms for the same reason they take warm baths. Heat relaxes muscles from the outside in. It allows for a greater range of motion in the ligaments, joints, and muscles. Capillaries — the extremely small vessels in body tissue that transport blood from the arteries to the veins — dilate in the heat, which helps deliver oxygen to tissue and muscles.

Exercising in heat also offers some subtle benefits:

- ✔ The heat may force you to slow down and do the exercises safely.
- ✔ Your heart beats faster to cool down your body, and this stimulated circulation speeds up body metabolism.
- ✔ The increased circulation and pumping action of your heart breaks down glucose and fat.
- ✔ The heat gives you a cardiovascular workout.
- ✔ The heat cleanses your body as you eliminate toxins through sweat.

Doing yoga with weights in a heated room sounds like a good deal. Stretching is a vital part of yoga with weights, and the heat helps you stretch. And the other benefits of exercising in a heated room aren't too shabby, either. You should run to your exercise area and turn up the thermostat immediately, right? The answer is: maybe. Exercising in a heated room has disadvantages, too.

Different people have different reactions to heat. Some of the reactions are harmless quirks:

- ✔ You may get very uncomfortable when sweat pours down your back and your heart starts beating faster.
- ✔ Sweat can be slippery on your yoga mat.
- ✔ The heat can keep you from relaxing, and relaxation is an essential part of the yoga frame of mind — a frame of mind that keeps you safe and growing in your practice.

Exercising in a heated room can also give you a case of lazy muscles. When a muscle gets too warm and relaxed, it can get lazy or groggy. It doesn't want to work anymore, and neither do you. If you've had the experience of sitting in a warm, comfortable bath and not wanting to ever get out, you know what lazy muscles are. You can find yourself stopping in the middle of a workout to use your yoga mat like a hammock rather than an exercise device.

Some reactions to heat are dangerous. Heat can add some unwelcome dimensions to the yoga practice:

- ✔ If you have high blood pressure, and you're concerned for the health of your heart, exercising in a hot room and cracking a profuse sweat can be frightening. Avoid exercising in the heat if the health of your heart is compromised or if you suspect in any way that exercising in the heat is bad for your health.

Consult your doctor before you decide to heat your exercise area if these thoughts enter your head.

✔ If you put an emphasis on pushing yourself further every time you exercise, you may do more harm than good in a heated environment. More is not always better, especially when it comes to your joints. Because warmer muscle tissue yields more easily, you run the risk of stretching beyond optimal limits and compromising joint tissue. A loose joint that you overstretch is like a loose door hinge that prevents the door from closing tightly and fitting in the frame.

Exercising in heat pushes you to the edge, and some people like being there. In our experience, certain type-A personalities who like getting their adrenalin and endorphins flowing enjoy the extra challenge of exercising in hot rooms. However, exercising gung-ho style can get you in trouble. When you exercise, always work to your capacity without compromising the stability and integrity of your joints, connective tissue, and muscles. Going at it full bore in a hot room makes it harder to maintain the mindfulness and awareness that yoga with weights calls for.

Still, some like it hot. If you're that kind of person, and you don't have health concerns, go ahead and raise the room temperature to 85 or 90°F. But remember that it isn't necessary to go that high to have a good yoga-with-weights workout; you can push yourself with 70 to 75°F just fine.

Don't expose yourself to drafts or a cold room when you exercise, because the cold air makes your muscles contract.

Jazzing up your workout with music

You may remember exercise programs from the 1980s that featured aerobic workouts accompanied by upbeat music. The idea was for the music to motivate you to exercise harder and to help you keep a tempo. These programs introduced many people to the concept of exercising to music. Thanks to modern portable music players, you can take your music with you when you exercise. It seems that half of all joggers have portable music players attached to their arms or waists. Half of all gym goers are also wired for sound.

It's up to you to decide whether you want to listen to music as you do your yoga-with-weights workouts. As the saying goes, music calms the wild beast. It can relax you, inspire you, motivate you, empower you, or rev you up, depending on your state of mind and what type of music you're listening to. In terms of yoga with weights, music can

✔ Help you set a pace for your workout

✔ Inspire you to keep going

✔ Comfort you when you're struggling with a difficult exercise

Meeting the challenge of exercising on your own

If you're the kind of person who likes to exercise on your own, or if you can't find yoga instructors where you live, you face additional challenges when exercising with yoga with weights. Here are some tips to help you on your way:

✔ **Take your time.** Nobody gets it right the first time. Take your time to understand what you're supposed to do in each exercise. Fortunately for you, yoga is an intuitive discipline. Nine times out of ten, you can "feel it" when you're doing an exercise right. You can feel the muscle groups at work and understand how each exercise is supposed to challenge you.

✔ **Start with warm-ups.** In a yoga-with-weights exercise class, instructors never neglect the warm-up phase of a workout, but people exercising at home often skip the warm-ups because they want to jump right in. Chapter 6 explains how to warm up for the exercises.

✔ **Practice the exercises without the weights initially.** Mastering many of the exercise forms is hard enough without having to lift the weights as well. After you understand

how to do an exercise, strap on the ankle weights and grab the hand weights.

✔ **Use a mirror.** The first few times you do an exercise, do it slowly and watch yourself in the mirror. See the section "Exercising in front of a mirror" earlier in this chapter for advice about what to look for when you exercise before a mirror. Try to make your reflection in the mirror look like the exercise photographs in this book.

✔ **Read this book carefully.** You are your best teacher and guide. You have wisdom and intelligence within you, and you have to tap your inner resources. In the end, because no instructor can tell you whether you're doing an exercise correctly, it's up to you to understand how to do an exercise and get the most out of it. That means reading this book more carefully than you would normally read an exercise book.

✔ **Record your voice reading the exercises aloud, and play back the recording as you exercise.** This gives you the illusion that you're in an exercise class and spares you from having to interrupt an exercise to consult this book.

However, music can also be a distraction. Throughout the exercises in this book, we ask you to "listen to your body" — to feel your muscles and ligaments as they stretch or contract so you can exert just the right amount of pressure and effort. If you introduce music into your yoga-with-weights workout, it can

✔ Prevent you from hearing your body and the sound of your breath

✔ Speed up the tempo of an exercise so you move too quickly

✔ Keep you from focusing and working out safely

If you prefer to exercise to musical accompaniment, ask yourself from time to time in the middle of a workout whether the music is a distraction. If it isn't a distraction, enjoy it for all its worth. Experiment with different kinds of music to find recordings that help you work out. We know people who listen to sounds from nature — ocean waves and babbling brooks — when they exercise; others love a good rhythm and beat. Any recording that deepens your yoga-with-weights workout is okay with us.

Working Out in a Group Setting

As of this writing, yoga with weights is a relatively new discipline. You can't walk into any yoga studio and ask to meet the yoga-with-weights instructor, because the studio may not have one — yet. We expect yoga with weights to become a popular exercise discipline in the years to come because it draws from deep tradition and rich experience in yoga and weightlifting. However, if you want instruction apart from what you can get from this book right away, you'll have to make do by finding an athletic trainer or yoga instructor. This part of the chapter helps you do just that. We give you tips on finding the right instructor, finding an affordable class, and practicing proper yoga etiquette.

Getting help from an athletic trainer or yoga instructor

Your yoga-with-weights workout can benefit from the help of an athletic trainer (also called a personal trainer). As little as an hour or two of instruction from a trainer can teach you the basics of weight training and show you the basic postures, even if the trainer doesn't have a background in yoga. The trainer can show you how to lift weights so you get a good workout without injuring yourself.

Similarly, a yoga instructor can help you with the basic yoga poses, even if he or she hasn't been trained in yoga with weights. Some poses we include in the exercises in this book, such as the warrior (shown in the Warrior I; Chapter 8), the downward-facing dog (shown in the Dog to Plank; Chapters 8 and 10), and the tree (shown in the Tree; Chapter 11), come straight from traditional yoga practices.

We recommend finding a certified and experienced yoga instructor, but if you can't find one, don't fret. Any high-quality yoga class that inspires you will help with your yoga-with-weights exercises because you discover the basics of aligning your body and breathing. When you go home to practice the exercises in this book, you'll have a better understanding of yoga mechanics.

Don't hesitate to show this book to your yoga instructor. If he or she is adventurous, your instructor may take an interest in yoga with weights. Yoga and fitness instructors often look for new, worthwhile exercise techniques that they can fold into their repertoires. If your instructor decides to take on yoga with weights, you may be able to come along for the ride. Who knows? Maybe you'll get a "finder's fee" and not have to pay for your lessons.

Finding the right instructor for you

People ask us all the time, "How do I find a good yoga instructor?" We can't give a simple answer to this question because there are so many different yoga schools, and every instructor is different. No single yoga teacher or yoga school is suitable for everyone. You have to find an instructor who fits your personality and meets your health goals.

Start your search for a good instructor by finding out if the teacher is certified. No single governing body certifies yoga instructors, and you can obtain a certificate with as little as a two-week training course, so receiving certification doesn't mean an instructor is necessarily qualified to teach yoga. But, generally speaking, a certified instructor is better than one who isn't certified. Being certified at least demonstrates a desire to learn about yoga and how to teach it to others.

The best way to investigate a teacher is to judge for yourself. Take a class from a teacher whose style appeals to you. Here are some questions to ponder as you decide whether an instructor is right for you:

- **Did you feel safe in the class?** A good teacher is mindful of his or her students' experience level and doesn't ask students to do exercises beyond their abilities.

- **Did the teacher offer modifications to the exercises?** Good teachers offer simpler, modified versions of exercises if they suspect or notice that students in the class can't do an exercise. This way, students can get some of the benefits of the exercise without putting themselves at risk for an injury. A good teacher can give guidance to advanced and beginning students at the same time.

- **Did the teacher give modifications without directing the instructions to a specific person?** A good teacher makes everyone feel at home. Except in praise, calling attention to a single person is inconsiderate. It makes the student feel self-conscious and takes away from his or her ability to do yoga exercises.

- **Did the teacher ask if any new students were in class?** Good teachers want to know their students' backgrounds so they can tailor their instructions accordingly. When teachers ask if new students are in class, it shows that they want to meet their students' needs.

> ✔ **Did the teacher appear to have eyes in the back of his or her head?**
> Good teachers seem to know what's going on in all parts of the room, whether there are 3 or 30 students.

No teacher is right for everyone. Get a reference from a friend or health practitioner, and then go and see for yourself. Different people have different personalities and are attracted to different schools of yoga and different yoga instructors. Some like grueling workouts in heated rooms so they fall in puddles of sweat when the classes are over. Others like to leave classes in advanced states of relaxation and repose. Trust your instincts and intuition when you choose a yoga teacher.

When you attend a class for the first time, introduce yourself to the teacher before class begins. Tell the teacher whether you have any special needs, whether you have injuries, if you're pregnant, and what your background in yoga is.

Considering the cost of taking yoga classes

How much a yoga class costs depends on what part of the country you're in. Classes range between $10 and $20 a session. Most yoga studios offer a package of five, ten, or more classes. Buying the classes in a package lowers the cost of the individual lessons. Classes run for 60, 75, or 90 minutes. Every studio is different, so to find information on sessions, packages, and so on, contact your local studio over the phone or on the Web.

Some health clubs have started offering yoga classes. If you're a member of a club that offers classes, you may be able to attend without paying more than your monthly membership fee. If you aren't a member of a club, look for health clubs that offer yoga classes. If your club doesn't offer the classes, nag the manager about it . . . well, "nag" isn't the right word. Try cajoling or persuading the manager to offer yoga classes.

Another way to find a bargain is to look into yoga studios in your area to see if they offer any workshops. Typically, master teachers run workshops, and they focus on one area of the body or one type of training. A weekend workshop may run two hours in the morning and two hours in the afternoon. Some workshops run over several weeks, and you attend the classes on the same day each week. Workshops are usually more rigorous in part because they last longer than standard classes, but also because they focus on a theme and give you a more thorough, in-depth practice experience. An intensive workshop can take you to the next level in your practice if you're ready and have a good experience.

Yoga workshops cost a minimum of $15 to $25 an hour, which is more than standard lessons, but the instruction is more focused and organized. Workshops and retreats give participants the chance to experience longer, extended instruction. Trainings serve to educate you on the study of posture and the philosophy of yoga.

Brushing up on your yoga-with-weights etiquette

If Miss Manners were a yoga instructor, she would want you to observe these fine points of yoga-with-weights etiquette:

- **Respect the yoga tradition.** Be mindful of others and of the yoga tradition when you enter the exercise room. Yoga classes are different from fitness classes in that most instructors prefer a quiet, contemplative atmosphere in the room.

- **Respect the silence.** As much as you want to ask a question of your instructor from time to time, try to wait until class is finished. Only one voice should be heard in the classroom — the teacher's. Remember that other students are concentrating on their workouts and on how their bodies feel, and they're listening carefully to the instructor's words — you should be, too. Asking a question in class may break the other students' concentration and disturb the flow of the class.

- **Don't arrive late.** Arriving late to any appointment is rude, but in yoga classes it's also a matter of safety. The first few exercises in a yoga class are meant to warm you up physically and mentally for the later exercises. If you skip the warm-up exercises, you may subject yourself to injury later on. Some instructors believe you should skip the class if you arrive more than five minutes late.

- **Don't leave early.** Some people have a "What's next?" mentality. They can't focus on the present because they're always looking ahead to their next activities. This kind of thinking runs contrary to the yoga philosophy, which says you should always be aware of the present and what you're doing in the here and now. Even if you're eager to go to your next appointment, don't leave class early.

- **Don't snap your mat open.** Admittedly, this is a pet peeve with us, but too many students snap their yoga mats open when they place them on the floor, and the noise disturbs others. It sounds like a giant rubber band snapping.

- **Leave your shoes and other belongings at the back of the room.** Practically speaking, if students litter their shoes and belongings around the room, it makes for an untidy and distracting mess. Leave your personal stuff in the back where others don't have to look at it. Spiritually speaking, you symbolically leave the world outside when you leave your belongings in the back of the room. You let go of outside distractions and say to yourself, "This is my time to focus on myself and my body."

✓ **Be careful with the weights.** Place the weights parallel to the floor so they don't tip over and fall on anyone. And never drop the weights. In old-style weightlifting, lifters dropped the weights on the floor when they finished the exercises. To keep from making too much noise, harming the floors, annoying the neighbors below, and hurting your toes, gently place the weights on the floor in a place where no one will step on them.

✓ **Deal with flatulence.** As we explain in Chapter 1, many yoga exercises fall in the squeeze-and-soak category, which means they massage your internal organs. This is good for you because the exercises squeeze toxins from your body, but they sometimes produce an unwanted side effect — flatulence. Usually the culprits are newcomers to the class, so be warned when newcomers start to twist and turn, especially if their mats are next to yours. Because deep breathing is an essential part of yoga with weights, and because the doors and windows are usually closed in exercise rooms, flatulence can be a real problem. As instructors, we're sometimes tempted to comment on flatulence to relieve the tension of having a silent-but-deadly killer in the room, but we don't want to embarrass the perpetrator, so we remain silent.

You can help prevent flatulence by not eating in the hour or two before class, avoiding foods that trigger flatulence in your body, and chewing your food slowly and carefully. After you gain experience and get healthier through regular exercise and a conscious choice of foods, excessive, uncontrollable flatulence usually diminishes.

✓ **Don't wear scents.** Many people are sensitive to fragrances, no matter how lovely or natural those fragrances purport to be. Remember that you're part of a group when you attend class. Come smelling as Mother Nature intended you to smell — fresh and clean, with no added fragrance. Everyone will breathe a sigh of relief.

Part I
Getting Started

The 5th Wave   By Rich Tennant

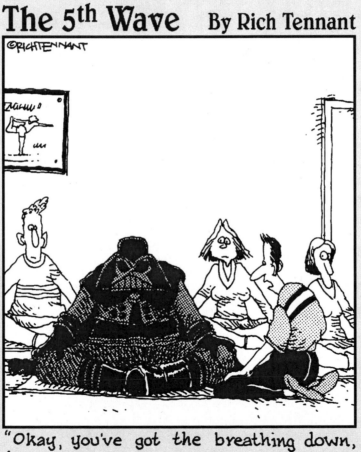

"Okay, you've got the breathing down, but wouldn't you be more comfortable in a different workout suit?"

In this part . . .

Part I is where you get your feet wet. Don't be shy. Walk right up to the shore and stick your toes in the water. We're here to show you the way.

In this part, you find out what yoga with weights is and all the different ways this exercise program can help you physically, mentally, and spiritually. We describe in detail the equipment you need for yoga with weights, and we show you how to get ready for your first workout. We also look at safety issues, show you how to manage exercise pain, and explain how to set up the ideal place for a yoga-with-weights workout.

Chapter 4

A Breath of Fresh Air: Yoga Breathing Techniques

*Y*our first and last acts on earth are one and the same — taking a breath. Your breath is with you at the very beginning and it will be with you until the very end. Breathing, you could say, is the most important activity you do. You can live for days without water and weeks without food, but only a few moments without breathing. Breath is your most intimate friend in life. You connect with the world around you most intimately not only by touch, sight, and hearing but also by breathing. The Sanskrit word for "life force," *prana* (pronounced *prah-nah*), is the same as the word for "breath."

This chapter explores why yoga breathing is so good for you and how it can benefit you during a yoga-with-weights workout. We also offer seven vibrant breathing techniques that will relax and revitalize you and that you can carry with you for the rest of your life.

Many people who study yoga report that the most practical lessons they learn from their studies are not only how to exercise and meditate, but also how to breathe in new and conscious ways that change their lives for the better. Before you read this chapter, take a breath and notice how you feel. Notice the air going in and out of your lungs and how the air feels in your nose, mouth, and throat. By the time you finish reading this chapter, you may breathe differently. The breath you're taking now could be one of the last you take in the old way.

Exploring the Breath-Mind Connection

You hear people say that when you get frustrated or angry you should "take a deep breath and count to ten." We can't vouch for the counting to ten part, but taking a deep breath is an excellent piece of folk wisdom. Deep breathing really can calm your nerves. It can relax and center you. Some people can even control the amount of pain they feel with breathing techniques. This ability is one of the reasons why, in prenatal clinics, expectant mothers study breathing techniques to control and help ease the pain of childbirth.

Breathing affects your state of mind, and for that reason, you can use breathing techniques that are supportive in cultivating a different state of mind. After you try these techniques, you may be delighted to find that you can change the mood you're in by breathing consciously and by paying attention to how you breathe. Your brain requires more oxygen than most other parts of your body. Supply it with the oxygen it needs to get more clarity of thought and to be able to concentrate for longer periods of time. Better breathing also affects your overall well-being. You get a greater sense of control over your happiness. In short, you feel more grounded and happier. You're more awake to the world around you and keener to enjoy that world.

To explore and experience a yoga-with-weights workout to the highest degree, we encourage you to focus on the sensations of your breathing. The mind doesn't wander as much if you establish a deep and rhythmic breath. When you catch your mind wandering (and it will wander), you can pull it back to the exercises by concentrating on your breath. Look at it this way: Imagine that your wandering mind is like a boat being pulled out to sea by the tide, but the boat is secured to a rope you hold in your hands. As the boat is floating away, you gently pull it back one breath at a time until your thoughts come back home to your body.

Besides helping you focus, conscientious breathing has an added benefit — it makes your workout safer. In weight training, many injuries take place due to repetitive stress; improper alignment; and throwing the weight around, which aggravates joints, tendons, and muscles. If you're distracted, preoccupied, or lackadaisical when you work out, you invite injury. Watch a person who has a great yoga-with-weights practice, and you notice his or her intense level of commitment and concentration. You see this person breathing in a deep and real way. Breathing helps you concentrate on your body so you know precisely how much effort and strength to put into the exercises without hurting yourself. The self-awareness that comes with conscientious breathing can actually help prevent injuries.

Considering the Health Benefits of Yoga Breathing

Besides benefiting your mental outlook (a topic we explore in the previous pages of this chapter), employing yoga breathing techniques offers many benefits to your health. Here are a handful of them:

- **Metabolism.** Breathing well, as nature intended, is supportive to the function of the digestive, respiratory, circulatory, and hormonal systems. Yoga breathing may be helpful in promoting your metabolic balance in everyday living. It may keep your body weight in check.

- **Detoxification.** Your lungs are a critical aspect of your daily detoxification. When you exhale, you release carbon dioxide that has been passed from your bloodstream into your lungs. Carbon dioxide is a waste product of your body's natural metabolism. By expelling air from the deepest recesses of your lungs, you expel more carbon dioxide and you enable your lungs to take in more oxygen.

- **Oxygenation.** One of the greatest benefits of yoga breathing is the oxygenation of all the cells in your body. The supply of oxygen to your brain and the muscles of your body increases. Oxygen travels the bloodstream by attaching to the hemoglobin in red blood cells. This oxygen enables your body to metabolize vitamins, minerals, and other nutrients. You get a lot of the same benefits from yoga breathing that you can get from visiting an oxygen bar, but you get them for free.

- **Organ massage.** Each time you inhale, your diaphragm descends and your abdomen expands (your diaphragm is a muscle located a few inches above your belly button; your abdomen is located over your belly). This action massages your intestines, heart, and other organs near your diaphragm. Proper breathing helps to promote improved circulation in these organs. What's more, it helps to strengthen and tone your abdominal muscles.

- **Posture.** The breathing techniques encourage good posture. Poor posture can be a cause of incorrect breathing.

According to the yoga tradition, each person is allotted a certain number of breaths, and after you exceed this number, your time on earth is finished. People who breathe hurriedly and shallowly use up their allotment of breaths quickly, but if you breathe slowly and consciously, your breath allotment lasts for many years. Let this thoughtful idea remind you how valuable and life-expanding each breath may be. Developing a breath that's balanced, steady, and rhythmic — one that's never forced but deep and full — helps you live a long and healthy life.

Practicing Yoga Breathing Techniques

The breathing techniques we present here are designed to relax and energize you. We didn't invent these breathing techniques; they're ancient practices from traditional yoga. The breath is the bridge between the mind and body. In traditional yoga, subtle breathwork and diaphragmatic breathing are helpful in leading you toward deeper self-realization. The breathing techniques are considered an art and science in the yoga system, and yoga teachers have skillfully refined and perfected these breathing techniques over the centuries.

You can practice these breathing techniques by themselves or as you do your yoga-with-weights workouts. You can consider these techniques "explorations." As you master these breathing techniques, pay attention to the subtle and sometimes powerful ways that they affect your body and mind. Get to know each technique so that you can call on it when you need it. For example, depending on how the techniques make you feel, you may try the Complete Breath when you're anxious or the Ocean Breath when you're low on energy. You can do these breathing techniques while you're sitting, lying down, or standing.

After experimenting for a while, you discover the breath that feels best to you while you're working out. For each workout in this book, we suggest a certain breath, but that doesn't mean you can't substitute a breath you prefer.

Following a few guidelines

No matter which breathing technique you undertake, follow these basic breathing guidelines:

- ✔ **Breathe through your nose unless we tell you to breathe through your mouth.** Breathing this way encourages you to breathe correctly and slowly because you can't force as much air through your nostrils as you can your mouth. Nostril breathing slows the process down. It also helps to filter and warm the air as it enters your body.

- ✔ **Listen to yourself breathe.** Does your breathing have a smooth and easy rhythm? Breathing is akin to the sound and rhythm of ocean waves — it's a natural act that changes pace with your moods and health. The breath is the link between the mind and the body. By listening to your breathing, you begin to control your breathing, and, in turn, you notice that you can gently shift your mood or disposition in subtle ways. Working gently with the sound and the sensations of your breath, you can subtly control how your body feels.

- ✔ **Breathe rhythmically.** If your breath stops or sounds rough, short, or shallow, it's a sign that you may be pushing too hard as you exercise. Forcing your breath suggests that you have come to the edge and gone in a bit too far. If your breath feels forced, take two or three Complete Breaths (which we explain in the section "The Complete Breath" later in this chapter) to get your rhythm and control back.

✔ **Concentrate on making a smooth transition between each inhalation and exhalation — focus on the point of stillness where one becomes the other.** Don't hold your breath at the top of an inhalation; ride it a bit over the top and then smoothly turn it into an exhalation. At the bottom of an exhalation, ride it out just a bit as well, and then smoothly transition into a natural inhalation.

✔ **Never force your breath beyond the natural capacity of your lungs.** Full, rhythmic, gentle breathing without strain is the goal of yoga breathing.

✔ **Don't practice yoga breathing in uncomfortable places where the air is too cold or too hot.** Like Goldilocks' porridge, the air should be "just right." Find a place that feels comfortable to you.

✔ **Straighten your posture.** If you slouch, let your belly hang out, round your shoulders, or stand without distributing and balancing the weight of your body properly, you can't possibly breathe well. If your posture is poor, you're crowding or collapsing your lungs and diminishing their capacity to take in oxygen. Lucky for you, the yoga-with-weights exercises in this book can improve your posture, and the combination of the exercises and the breathing techniques can significantly increase the amount of nourishing oxygen you take into your body.

The Complete Breath

The Complete Breath is a wonderful breath to live your life with — it's the basis of all other breathing techniques and is at the very heart of yoga-with-weights exercises. The Complete Breath engages your entire respiratory system. Besides raising and gently opening your collarbone and rib cage area, you engage your abdomen evenly and activate your diaphragm naturally, thus creating a full and deep breath.

The Complete Breath is a great way to relieve tension and stress. It improves the quantity and quality of the oxygen that enters your body. It helps your body find its balance and energy to live life. In times of stress, the Complete Breath helps to combat shortness of breath and calm your nervous system. Practice the Complete Breath when you feel angry, impatient, or nervous.

Ideally, you should inhale and exhale six times per minute when using the Complete Breath. Breathing through your nostrils, you inhale four to six counts at minimum, and you exhale six to ten counts at minimum. Of course, this is the ideal, but if you're new to yoga with weights, inhale as many counts as you can without straining, and try to reach the four- to six-count minimum.

Follow these steps to perform the Complete Breath:

1. **While sitting, lying down, or standing, relax your shoulders and gaze straight ahead or close your eyes.**

   Your mouth and jaw should be relaxed, your windpipe should feel open, and your chin should be pointing gently down. Make sure your back is erect but not rigid.

2. **Inhaling slowly through your nose, feel your abdomen, your mid-body (the diaphragm area), and your upper chest gently expand until you fill your lungs to capacity.**

   Notice the breathing sensation everywhere, but especially in your upper chest first. Feel your diaphragm moving calmly. Allow your ribs and chest to remain soft, open, and relaxed.

3. **Exhaling slowly through your nose, gently engage your abdomen.**

   Feel your body and your diaphragm gently coming back to center as you empty your lungs.

Practice the Complete Breath ten times, inhaling to a count of four and exhaling to a count of six.

Try taking the Complete Breath a step further by expanding your abdomen as you inhale and feeling your rib cage expand as you fill your lungs to the brim with air, as if you're inflating a balloon. Begin to exhale by drawing your belly in and up. Feel the sides of your ribs pressing or squeezing back in like a bellows or accordion as you empty your lungs and allow your chest to relax. Continue to breathe in this fashion for a minute or two.

Never force your lungs to inhale or expel air. Feel your lungs filling evenly and calmly in all directions — up, down, into each side, forward, and back. As you take Complete Breaths, see whether, by directing your attention there, you can inflate and awaken sensations in the sides and back of your body as well as in the front of your body. Practice in each area by isolating it first with your mind and then directing your breath into each area for one, two, or three breaths.

The Abdominal Breath

Do the Abdominal Breath when you're feeling tension, stress, or fatigue. This breath relaxes you. A few minutes of deep abdominal breathing can help bring greater connectedness between your mind and your body. In essence, the goal is to shift from upper chest, short, shallow breathing to deeper abdominal breathing. Concentrate on your breath and try to breathe in and out gently through your nose. With each breath, allow any tension in your body to slip away. After you start breathing slowly with your abdominals, sit quietly and enjoy the sensation of physical relaxation.

Follow these steps to practice the Abdominal Breath:

1. **Lie on your back or sit comfortably in a chair.**

2. **Place one hand on your abdomen just above your pubic bone and below your navel; place your other hand on your solar plexus right beneath your breastbone.**

3. **Listening to your breath, inhale slowly and deeply through your nostrils — so deeply that your belly expands and you feel a wave of breath moving into the bottom, or lowest recesses, of your lungs.**

   Get down to the bottom of your lungs with this inhalation, going as low and as deep inside your lungs as you can. You can feel the rounding of your abdomen in your hands such that your hands rise a bit and your abdominal cavity pushes upward. Meanwhile, your chest opens and expands gently as if your abdomen is a balloon filling with air evenly and equally in all directions.

4. **At the top of your inhalation, find the point of transition where the inhale becomes an exhale.**

   At the top of every breath is a point of passage, the place where the inhale ends and the exhale begins. Find that place within your lungs and pause a moment to notice how your breath gently begins to shift in a new direction.

5. **To a count of six to eight (or more) seconds, exhale fully through your nostrils.**

   Feel your whole body releasing tension and letting go. Allow your body, including your arms and legs, to relax and go limp.

Do ten slow, full Abdominal Breaths.

Try to breathe smoothly and regularly without gasping for breath or letting your breath out all at once. Let each exhalation roll out like a long, slow ocean wave. Remember to notice that transition, or turning point, at the end of each inhalation and exhalation when one becomes the other in a seamless transition. If you can manage it, try to get in a rhythm and practice the Abdominal Breath for 10 minutes.

The Abdominal Breath is _very_ relaxing. It really works when done well, and for that reason, you may not want to practice it while you're driving. One of Sherri's students missed her freeway turnoff by three exits because she practiced Abdominal Breathing behind the wheel of her car. She was able to induce such a deep state of relaxation during her journey that she forgot her reason for driving her car. Be careful and, along with driving safely, breathe wisely.

If your breathing becomes too rapid, short, or shallow, you may start hyperventilating. And hyperventilating, in turn, sometimes can cause symptoms similar to those of a panic attack. Hyperventilating occurs when you breathe out too much carbon dioxide relative to the amount of oxygen in your bloodstream. If you find that your breathing is shallow and you're breathing in an anxious way, try taking an Abdominal Breath. Taking Abdominal Breaths helps you shift into deeper, more rhythmic breathing.

The Ocean Breath

The Ocean Breath — sometimes called "rib breathing" or the "upward-moving breath" — oxygenates your blood. It stimulates your circulation and gives you a burst of energy. This dynamic breath awakens you and brings you into the present moment. It's also a warming breath.

You emit a sound during the Ocean Breath — the sound (you guessed it) of an ocean breeze. You stay in your chest and fill your lungs from the diaphragm upward. To stay inflated, your lungs rely on a vacuumlike action inside your chest, and then you push out a full, deep, and complete exhalation through your nostrils. This breath is different from the Complete Breath (which we explain earlier in this chapter) because you mostly engage your chest and rib cage, and you gently contract your abdomen.

Follow these steps to practice the Ocean Breath:

1. **Stand or sit comfortably with your spine straight.**

2. **Place your arms on your chest with the fingers of your right hand tucked into your left armpit and the fingers of your left hand tucked into your right armpit.**

3. **Close your eyes or gaze straight ahead with your windpipe open, your jaw and mouth relaxed, and your chin pointing gently downward.**

4. **Inhale to a count of six to ten, engaging the sipping muscles in the back of your throat as if you're sipping through a straw, and feel your ribs opening and your breath filling to the top of your lungs.**

   Inhale to whichever count you can manage best.

   Pay attention to the tip of your nose as you inhale. It enhances the sensation of filling your chest all the way up.

5. **Gently, but with some commitment and determination, exhale steadily through your nostrils until the exhale is complete.**

   Feel your breath passing from the back of your throat, across the roof of your mouth, and out your nostrils. You hear a hissing sound, something similar to the sound of a hose when you turn it on and the water begins rushing out.

Never push too hard; this breath is dynamic, but never forced. Feel yourself releasing the air. When you push the air out, your abdominal muscles come into play a bit more. The exhale is something like a volcanic eruption that begins at the diaphragm and rises with increasing strength.

Take 10 Ocean Breaths; pause to rest; do 10 more; pause to rest again; and if you like the results, do 10 more for a total of 30 breaths. Then you can let your abdomen relax and your breath normalize once again.

Perfecting the Ocean Breath takes time, especially when you try smoothing out the transition between inhaling and exhaling, but stick with it. As yoga teachers say, "Breath into breath, moment into moment."

 As you get better at the Ocean Breath, you may begin to notice a subtle sensation, or tingling, in your spine. This subtle sensation begins in the base or bottom of your spine and moves gently upward. When you exhale, you may experience the gentle sensation of your breath moving downward, even though the air is leaving your throat and nose. See whether you can detect these two sensations — the tingling in your spine moving upward and your breath moving downward — meeting in your solar plexus. Try to feel the breath inside the breath. When the two sensations merge, you may experience an awakened inner consciousness and an overall sense of well-being.

The Balancing Breath

The object of the Balancing Breath is to develop a conscious control of your breathing. Try this simple breathing technique when you feel tired or overwhelmed or when you just want to clear your head for a moment. The Balancing Breath is similar to the Complete Breath (which we cover earlier in this chapter), except that you inhale and exhale to a count of four instead of exhaling for a longer period of time.

Follow these steps to practice a Balancing Breath:

1. **Sit, lie down, or stand with your shoulders, mouth, and jaw relaxed.**

   Your choice: Gaze softly straight ahead or close your eyes. Make sure your back is erect but not rigid.

2. **To a count of four, slowly inhale through your nose.**

   Feel your breath expanding into your abdomen, mid-body (the diaphragm area), and upper chest. Without forcing, engage and gently fill your lungs to their full capacity.

3. **To a count of four, exhale slowly through your nose, drawing your abdomen gently in and up to help send the breath smoothly out.**

Although your breath empties from your lungs, focus on releasing it first with your abdomen, and then with your diaphragm, and then with your upper chest. Emit all the air from your lungs.

Practice the Balancing Breath six to ten times — inhaling to a count of four and exhaling to a count of four — pause to rest for a moment, and then do another six to ten Balancing Breaths.

As you begin to perfect the Balancing Breath, consider inhaling to eight counts and exhaling to eight counts.

You can also inhale for four counts, hold the inhalation very softly for four counts, and then exhale completely for four counts. Try to find a rhythm as you do this variation on the Balancing Breath. Make your breath roll in like a wave; hold softly so your lungs can drink in the oxygen; and gently exhale all the air.

The Alternate Nostril Breath

In the Alternate Nostril Breath, you breathe through one nostril at a time, switching off from breath to breath (sorry, you can't do this one if you're congested or have a stuffy nose). You may be surprised by how you feel as you take Alternate Nostril Breaths. The breath offers many physical and subtle benefits. Each nostril is associated with one cerebral brain hemisphere. The right nostril is associated with the right brain hemisphere (where your spatial perceptions begin), and the left nostril is associated with the left brain hemisphere (where your verbal skills are). Breathing through alternate nostrils stimulates alternate brain hemispheres. In traditional yoga, the right nostril is considered the warming and energetic one, and the left nostril is considered the cool and calming one.

Practice the Alternate Nostril Breath to calm your mind and nervous system in times of stress. It induces a powerful sense of being in the present moment and increases your mental clarity and alertness.

Follow these steps to test-drive the Alternate Nostril Breath:

1. **Sit comfortably with your eyes closed.**

2. **Close your right nostril by pressing your nose gently with your right thumb, and then inhale through your left nostril to a count of four.**

   Feel your breath flowing into the open nostril. Notice if the air feels cool or warm. See how deeply into your body you can detect the breath. Do you feel it in your throat? The tops of your lungs? The bottoms?

3. **Close your left nostril by gently pressing with your right ring finger and pinky finger into your nose; at the same time, remove your thumb from your right nostril and exhale through your right nostril to a count of eight.**

Ideally, you want to exhale twice as long as you inhale.

Exhale quietly and evenly into the lower, middle, and upper regions of your lungs.

4. **Repeat the breath, but this time close your left nostril and inhale through your right to a count of four, and then close your right nostril and exhale to a count of eight through your left nostril.**

Start by doing six to ten complete Alternate Nostril Breath cycles. It requires five to eight minutes of concentrated breathing.

As you develop your technique, try inhaling and exhaling for longer periods of time, always keeping the 2-to-1 ratio of exhales to inhales. You should never force your breathing, but you can lengthen the inhale and exhale to longer counts as you develop your technique. For example, try inhaling for 8 counts and exhaling for 16 counts.

The Cleansing Breath

The purpose of the Cleansing Breath is to clean and clear out your lungs. This breath is unique, because instead of exhaling through your nose, you exhale through your mouth as you purse your lips. Pursing your lips creates pressure on your airways and helps keep them open so stale air can exit your lungs. It feels almost as though you're releasing pent-up emotions when you do the Cleansing Breath. In effect, you emit a "sigh of relief."

If you can, practice the Cleansing Breath outside in the fresh morning air. Follow these steps to practice a Cleansing Breath:

1. **Inhale a Complete Breath comfortably through your nostrils to the count of four to six.**

We explain the Complete Breath in the section "The Complete Breath" earlier in this chapter.

2. **Gently purse your lips as you strongly exhale to a count of four.**

Exhale vigorously so you make a loud whooshing sound. Feel your breath rising from the bottom to the top of your lungs in a dynamic and complete release. Refreshing, isn't it? You feel as though you're cleansing your entire system.

Gently contracting your abdominal muscles as you exhale helps push the air out.

Complete this breath four to six times.

The Vitality Breath

We saved the most dynamic breath for last. The Vitality Breath is a fantastic breath with which to start a yoga-with-weights workout. It sends energy to all parts of your body and makes you feel more alive.

Follow these steps to practice the Vitality Breath:

1. **Stand upright with your feet spread wider than your hips and your toes pointing forward.**

   Make sure your body weight is well-balanced between both legs.

2. **While inhaling a Complete Breath through your nostrils to the count of four, extend your arms straight out in front of you, palms facing upward.**

   This is the starting position.

   We explain the Complete Breath in the section "The Complete Breath" earlier in this chapter. Although you hold your arms in front of you, you should hold them in a relaxed manner.

3. **Exhale slowly through your mouth or through pursed lips as you draw your hands toward your body along the sides of your rib cage and gradually contract the muscles of your arms and hands.**

   By the time your arms and hands reach the sides of your body, contract your muscles so that your fists are clenched. Put some force into it. At this point, your fists should be tightly clenched and you should feel a driving force or sense of inner release as you exhale.

4. **Relax your arms and hands as you deeply inhale, slowly unclench your fists, and return to the starting position (see Step 2).**

   Imagine that you're taking in this breath through your hands and heart.

Repeat Steps 2 through 4 six to eight times to complete six to eight Vitality Breaths.

Keep it going. If you like the way the Vitality Breath feels, do two sets of six to eight breaths. Listen to the sound you make as you exhale. The Vitality Breath is a commanding exercise. Don't be shy about exploring this powerful, energy-enhancing breath, but if it doesn't feel right to you, just stay with the Complete Breath.

Chapter 5

Making the Mind and Body Connection

*Y*ou may not know it, but when you exercise, you have the potential to exercise with your mind as well as your body. And in yoga with weights, the mind plays a bigger part than it does in other exercise disciplines, because one of the goals of yoga with weights is to be self-aware and to develop your relationship with your consciousness in everything you do.

This chapter explores training your mind and some of the mental aspects of yoga with weights. You look into quieting and calming your mind, listening to your body as you exercise, and breaking the mental barriers that keep you from wanting to exercise. You also discover a mental visualization technique for focusing your mind and a special contract-and-release exercise for wringing all the tension from your body.

Taming the Monkey Mind

One of the objects of traditional yoga is to discover how to calm your mind to achieve clarity of thought. An overactive mind is sometimes called a "monkey mind." In traditional yoga, a monkey mind is one that swings wildly from branch to branch — that is, from thought to thought — without really considering where it's going. A monkey mind is always busy, so much so that it leaves you feeling exhausted and robs you of your precious energy resources and your ability to concentrate.

Taming a monkey mind isn't easy. It takes time, practice, and, perhaps most importantly, a commitment to discovering how to relax your mind and always remain in the moment. What does "in the moment" mean? It means to be consciously aware of your surroundings and how you feel *now* — not letting your mind drift into memories or fantasies. When you tame the monkey mind, you achieve self-awareness and the ability to think with clarity. You literally pull yourself together, body and mind. For more tips on taming a monkey mind, check out "Bringing Your Mind into the Present Moment" later in this chapter.

Focusing on the Transitions

Yoga masters pay a lot of attention to transitions. The entire yoga philosophy is not about abrupt stops and starts, but smooth transitions of breath into breath and moment into moment. This philosophy applies to all activities in life — the transition between sleep and wakefulness, the transition between work and play, and even the transition from year to year and decade to decade, for example. In yoga class, it means paying as much attention to getting into and out of a pose as being in the pose itself.

The object is to make all transitions, from the smallest to the largest, smooth and graceful so you maintain your self-awareness and your yoga consciousness as a matter of course, no matter what you do or where you go. When you take on a yoga lifestyle, you strive to make all your activities — all the moments of your life — one vast, inspired moment imbued with yoga consciousness. This effort gives you a greater sense of personal empowerment and freedom of choice as you skillfully live your life. With each breath and each moment leading one to the other, you're fully alive as you embrace your life to its fullest without missing out on a single moment of the journey.

Easier said than done, of course, but yoga with weights can help. To start down the road of greater consciousness, focus on the transition between yoga-with-weights exercises and how you link one breath to the next. (See Chapter 4 for breathing details.) Try to create effortless, flowing, graceful transitions between exercises, with as little excess movement as possible. That means when the mind wanders, as it will, you gently pull it back and focus on what you're doing in the present. When you forget to breathe properly, you put more mental effort into breathing next time. You observe your own training, and, in the process, you become your own peak-performance coach. No one knows better than you do whether you're getting the most out of yoga-with-weights exercises.

By focusing on the transitions between exercises, you can carry vitality, strength, and endurance from one exercise to the next. With enough attention to transitions, you can turn your yoga-with-weights workout into a living dance, with all the postures connected through balance, presence, attention, and breath. And guess what? You'll even have some fun in the process.

Exercising from the Inside Out

Yoga with weights is different from nearly all forms of exercise in that you do the exercises "from the inside out." In basketball and weightlifting, for example, the object is to do something outside of your body — make a basket or press a certain amount of weight. But in yoga with weights, the object of the exercises is found mostly within, not outside the body. Like all forms of yoga, yoga with weights is a profound technique for getting in touch with your body. As you perform an exercise, you feel and listen to the inner workings of your body. Your body tells you whether you're doing the exercise correctly, and part of your job is to discover how to listen. If you're in tune with yourself — if you feel balanced, if you feel the right combination of muscles at work, if you're pushing yourself precisely to the threshold of your ability — you'll know it.

Exercising from the inside out takes some getting used to for people who aren't accustomed to exercising this way. It requires a fair amount of patience; it requires you to focus within; and, to a certain degree, it requires you to rely on your intuition and to notice the subtle sensations in your body. Although instructors can help you with your posture and movements, knowing whether you're exercising correctly is ultimately up to you, and you'll know because you can feel it. No outside objective — jumping to a certain height, lifting a certain amount of weight — can tell you whether you're on target with an exercise. Only you, your intuition, your innate wisdom, and your intelligence can tell you when you're exercising right. Figuring it out may take some time, and it takes practice, but when you do, it feels great.

Letting Go of "I Can't Do It"

More so than muscle fatigue, what keeps most people from yoga with weights is that broken record that each person has in his or her record collection, the one that says over and over and over again, "You can't do it." Exercising is hard in and of itself; attempting a new exercise program may be even harder.

The only way to push aside "I can't do it" is to use your head. When the old record starts playing, take notice and then focus on your breathing. Listen to the air slowly entering and slowly leaving your lungs. This technique helps quiet your mind and keeps the record from playing. It helps you immerse yourself in the exercises. (For more information on breathing during yoga-with-weights exercises, see Chapter 4.)

Resistance to exercising can come from many different places. Everyone can find excuses not to exercise. Everyone can think of things they'd rather do. We've discovered that the easiest way to break through old barriers that your mind has built up against exercise is to take the first step or the first yoga breath. After you get going, you discover that exercising isn't as hard as you thought it was. Let each exercise session act as a new beginning and a fresh start. Take it one breath at a time. Make that your objective. Personal power — your greatest potential — rests within. When you bring what's within out into the world, miracles happen. (See Chapter 19 for motivational tips for yoga with weights.)

Bringing Your Mind into the Present Moment

Bringing your mind into the present moment is easier said than done. All people have distractions that keep them from focusing on the moment. To help you get there, we offer you a mental visualization technique and an exercise for relieving tension. Turn to these pages when you want to coax yourself into living in the present. In a way, we're asking you to live life to the fullest by being in the moment.

Visualizing a calmer mind

One way to tame a wild and overly active mind — a monkey mind (see "Taming the Monkey Mind" earlier in this chapter) — is visualization. *Visualization* is when you close your eyes and go on a mental journey as a means of calming your mind and achieving a quiet, meditative state of self-awareness. In effect, you become the producer of your own visual effects — a sort of director of your own mental movies. The idea is to reach a state of deep relaxation and focus.

The object of the following visualization is to discover a refuge of calm and quiet within yourself. You need at least 10 minutes for this visualization. Lights, camera, action:

1. **Lie down or sit comfortably in a quiet place.**

   Do your best to find a place where you aren't bothered by cell phones and other distractions.

2. **Notice the tip of your nose and the coolness or warmth of each breath as the stream of air flows in and out of your nostrils.**

3. **Keeping your attention on the tip of your nose, feel the sensations of your lungs as they fill with air and then empty themselves of air.**

   Focus on your lungs for at least six breaths.

4. **Imagine that the innermost center of your body, from your hips up to your shoulders, is a deep pond.**

5. **View this deep pond in your mind and direct your attention to the surface of the pond.**

6. **Notice the currents or waves on the surface of the pond and look toward the sky, above the pond in your mind, and observe any clouds.**

   The clouds represent your emotions, and the surface of the pond represents your thoughts. In the next several steps in the visualization, you sink deeper into the image of the pond and distance yourself from your flow of emotions and the activity of your thoughts.

7. **Visualize dropping a pebble into the pond.**

   In your mind, follow that pebble with all your awareness as it sinks deeper into the pond. Breathe in and out calmly and quietly, remaining aware of the tip of your nose if doing so helps you breathe more calmly and deeply.

8. **As the pebble continues to sink (which represents deeper levels of your awareness), feel a sense of your own depth, the calmness within you, and the stilling and quieting of your mind as the pebble falls into deeper waters of inner knowing.**

9. **Imagine the pebble coming to rest on the bottom of the pond.**

   You're at a point of restfulness in the depths; dwell here for as long as you want.

10. **In the role of an observer, step back from this visualization and notice that you've taken your mind and thoughts into deeper waters.**

   High above, the clouds (your emotions) are still alive and well, and the surface of the pond (your thoughts) is still ripe with currents and activity. Down in the depths, however, you are still and quiet. You've discovered the deeper well of a steady mind and calm deep within you. This state is known as *equanimity,* when the mind is calm and aware.

   Dwell comfortably and securely in this place of calm for as long as you care to remain. Remember: This place of calmness is always there waiting in case you need to visit it.

Releasing tension with a contract-and-release exercise

The object of this contract-and-release exercise is to release tension in your body and bring your mind into the present moment. You isolate different areas of your body one at a time, starting with your toes and working your way up to your head. In each body area, you contract your muscles hard and then gently relax them. The idea is to tense each muscle group hard, without straining, for about five to ten seconds, and then suddenly let go of the tension or contraction. When you release your muscles, you do so fully and abruptly, relaxing and letting your body fall completely limp. In this way, you achieve a state of deeper relaxation, and you systematically relieve tension from different areas of your body.

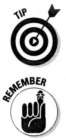

Visualize each muscle group you're working on in your mind's eye before you contract and relax the muscle group. By directing your thoughts into a part of your body, you can discover the nerve pathways necessary for relaxation. You discover how to relax by directing your mental energy toward your body.

Repeat the contract-and-release sequence three times with each part of your body you're working on. Hold the first contraction for five counts, the second for about seven, and the third for about ten. As you do so, inhale through your nose during contractions and exhale through pursed lips after you relax your muscles. Inhale deeply, yet not so deeply that you feel discomfort in your chest or lungs.

This exercise takes a bit of time — perhaps 10 to 20 minutes — but it's well worth the effort. Follow these steps to do the contract-and-release exercise:

1. **Lie down on your back in a quiet, comfortable place, and take a few deep, slow, Abdominal Breaths (Chapter 4 explains what these breaths are).**

   As you exhale, notice the weight of your body and how that weight is distributed on the carpet or on your yoga mat.

   In the next seven steps, starting with your toes and working upward, contract and relax muscle groups for five seconds.

2. **Direct your attention to your right and left legs and, in a wavelike action that moves from your feet upward, tighten your feet by curling your toes downward, and then relax.**

   If your muscles cramp, relax and gently shake off the cramp or wait until it stops, and then start again. Sometimes the muscles act up because you haven't used them in such a deep way for a while.

3. **Move the contractions up higher, tightening your calf muscles while flexing your toes toward you or turning your toes under (do whichever feels best).**

4. **Move the contraction higher again, engaging the muscles of your thighs all the way up to your hips.**

   You may tighten your buttocks along with your thighs, because the thigh muscles attach to that area. Feel your thigh muscles smoothing out and relaxing completely as you exhale.

5. **Tighten and relax your buttocks, hips, and abdominal areas.**

6. **Contract and release your back and chest.**

   As you relax, imagine a wave of release moving smoothly downward from your chest. Feel the excess tension in your chest flowing away with each exhalation.

7. **Clench your fists and feel the contraction moving up your arms; relax your arms and hands.**

   If you have to lift your arms from the floor, you can do so. Notice the muscles around your shoulder blades pushing in.

8. **Tense and relax the muscles in your neck, forehead, face, and scalp, as well as the muscles around your ears.**

   Be careful not to grind your teeth. Feel the frown lines on your face melting away.

9. **Repeat Steps 2 through 8, holding each muscle contraction for seven counts before releasing.**

10. **Repeat Steps 2 through 8 again, holding each muscle contraction for ten counts before releasing.**

11. **Take a deep, full breath and mentally scan your body for any tension that still remains; notice where you're still holding tight, and contract and relax the muscles there.**

    Feel your body resting deeply.

12. **Inhale and, as you gently hold your breath, contract your muscles everywhere — bottom to top, front to back, inside to outside, outside to inside, forward and back, up and down.**

    Feel a wave of contraction moving from your held breath into every area of your body.

13. **Exhaling quickly through your mouth, release all the muscles you've been contracting.**

    You'll hear a swooshing or deep-releasing *ahh* sound that rises from your belly as you exhale.

14. **Repeat Steps 12 and 13 three times.**

    Finish by resting gently. Let your breathing become natural again. Enjoy the sensations of your body resting on the floor.

Playing a bit of soothing music in the background helps some people with this exercise. And this exercise is a great way to finish off a yoga-with-weights workout!

Chapter 6

Warming Up and Cooling Down

....

In This Chapter

▶ Looking at the benefits of warming up

▶ Walking as a prelude to working out

▶ Doing the yoga-with-weights warm-up exercises

▶ Discovering how to meditate

▶ Using meditation to cool down after your workout

....

*T*his chapter focuses on warming up to get ready for a yoga-with-weights workout and cooling down when your workout is over. We show you the benefits of warming up, and you discover why simple activities such as walking can be such great warm-up techniques. And when you finish warming up and complete your yoga-with-weights workout, we show you how to pull all the elements of your exercise practice into a final meditation that will leave you feeling refreshed.

Don't let the word "meditation" intimidate you; it isn't as complicated as most people think. Meditation is the finishing touch, the icing on your workout cake — the part of the workout that serves as a peaceful and calming transition to the rest of your day.

Reaping the Benefits of Warming Up

Most people like to jump into the workout pool without getting their feet wet first. They want to start exercising without warming up. They want to get right to it, get the ball rolling, finish, and not look back. What they don't realize is that warming up has some real advantages, both physical and mental. You've heard it before: Warming up is recommended no matter what kind of exercise you intend to do. In yoga with weights, warming up is especially important, because yoga with weights works your muscles and joints more than other exercise programs.

What's that crackling sound?

When you stretch, you may hear a cracking sound in your joints and muscles. To see what we mean, try rolling your head from your chest to your shoulder to your back to your other shoulder and to your chest again. Do you hear a crackling noise?

What you're hearing is the sound of *synovial fluid* — the fluid found in joints and tendon sheaths — breaking up. The fluid acts as a kind of lubricant to enable your limbs to move in their sockets. When your joints are stiff, the synovial fluid gets stuck, but moving your joints and limbs breaks up the deposits. Over time, if you stick with yoga with weights, the excessive crackling noise starts to diminish along with the synovial fluid deposits, keeping things fluid and free in movement.

Here are some of the advantages of warming up:

- ✔ **Warming up helps prevent injuries.** Preparing your muscles, tendons, and ligaments makes them more flexible and less susceptible to injury. You ready them to perform the dynamic yoga-with-weights exercises that follow.

- ✔ **Warming up coaxes your body into flexibility.** It makes your body more supple and mobile. Your joints and muscles are better able to move through their full ranges of motion.

- ✔ **Warming up promotes a natural release of synovial fluid into the joints.** As we explain in the "What's that crackling sound?" sidebar, synovial fluid acts as a lubricant to cushion your joints and help make your limbs more flexible.

- ✔ **Warming up, like the exercises themselves, helps stimulate the flow of blood — and of oxygen — to your muscles.** This makes your body warmer and your muscles more pliable. In other words, you get a better workout.

- ✔ **Warming up slows you down and brings you into the moment.** You start to focus on moving your body, which prepares you for the full workout to come. In other words, being present mentally as you start gives you confidence to rock-and-roll right into the exercises.

Stretching is a process-oriented activity. It isn't about how far or how hard you stretch. Stretching is really about the journey and finding out how to coax your muscles into better and deeper stretches. You have to realize that to stretch a muscle, it must be relaxed.

Walking to Warm Up

Walking is the most natural of all exercises. It can also be one of the most — if not *the* most — enjoyable exercises. Walking doesn't require any particular expertise, either; it gives everyone the chance to be physically active.

If you have the time, make walking a prelude to every yoga-with-weights workout. You don't have to hike to the top of Mt. Everest — a short walk of 10 to 20 minutes will do. Getting in a walk daily or every other day has all kinds of benefits for your body and your mind. And if you combine walking with the other short warm-up exercises we describe in this chapter, you'll be well prepared for your yoga-with-weights workout. The combination of walking and yoga with weights as a daily and/or weekly workout program enhances the quality of your general health and mental well-being. It also helps keep your weight in check.

In the following pages, we explain the benefits of including a walk in your daily warm-up routine. We also explain how to walk properly to take stock of the world around you and the world inside you and how to prepare your body for a workout.

We recommend walking outside in nature, weather permitting. If you can't walk outside, a treadmill in your home or gym works well. Put all your walking clothes by the door so you're ready to get up and go before your workout. Because footwear is important, buy walking shoes that fit well (see Chapter 2 for some advice about buying walking shoes).

Fluids are essential if you want to take longer walks. Be sure to bring along water if you plan to walk for any length of time. (Chapter 2 looks into the particulars of staying hydrated as you exercise.)

Improving your mindfulness

If you decide to walk outside, you get a chance to look around and enjoy nature, of course, and you enjoy the benefits of performing a physical activity. Walking increases the oxygen to your brain and muscles, reduces stress, and slows bone mineral loss. The stimulus of seeing the world outside the confines of your house or office — and seeing the world move while you walk — calms your mind and body.

As you walk, be mindful of your breathing. Make your short walk a moving meditation by synchronizing your breathing with your steps. As you put one foot in front of the other, focus on the count of each breath. Take four counts to breathe in and four to breathe out. Being mindful of your breathing as you walk is good practice for being mindful of your breathing in your yoga-with-weights exercises and in everything you do. It also sharpens your awareness of breathing and increases your powers of concentration.

Breathe through your nostrils, or take Complete Breaths (Chapter 4 explains what those are). You can also try saying the following sentence silently with each breath to get into the four-count rhythm: "Breathing in I calm body and mind; breathing out I cleanse and clear."

Preparing for a workout

For the first five minutes of your walk, stroll in an easy manner with your head held in whatever position feels most comfortable. Find your natural stride, feel your feet connecting with the ground, and gaze straight ahead. Gradually start to pick up speed, but never walk so fast that you're uncomfortable or have to strain to catch your breath. If you're walking with a companion, you should be able to carry on a conversation without having to stop to catch your breath.

As you walk, swing your arms gently alongside your body in a natural arc. Notice the movement of your arms, and develop an opposite-arm, opposite-leg movement — in other words, a coordinated stride. Walk with purpose and direction. Feel your chest lift up and open, and feel the energy flowing through your body.

As you walk, you can burn more calories by increasing your pace or walking up and down hills. Just be careful not to overextend yourself. If you don't push too hard, you're more likely to exercise regularly.

Adding a Handful of Warm-Up Exercises to Your Walk

Along with walking to warm up (the subject of the previous section), you can do warm-up exercises. We describe these exercises in the pages that follow. These warm-ups will keep your juices flowing after your walk and lead you comfortably into your yoga-with-weights workout. None of these exercises is difficult. None takes more than a minute to complete. Feel free to do as few or as many of these warm-up exercises as you want before your workout.

Choose exercises that warm up the parts of your body that feel tight or stiff. You can also choose exercises that make you feel better or relax you and prepare you physically and mentally for the workout to come.

A skeptic may say that the warm-up exercises we present here are too easy and can't be of much help. Here are a few reasons why we firmly disagree:

✔ After you complete a few of these warm-up exercises, you'll notice that warming up makes a yoga-with-weights workout more productive.

✔ If you're not up to doing the actual yoga-with-weights exercises yet because you're too stiff, you can prepare your body by doing these warm-up exercises as a workout. They give beginners a fairly good workout until they feel comfortable enough to start with the exercises.

✔ If you feel sore the day after a yoga-with-weights workout, you can use these warm-up exercises to relieve discomfort. These warm-ups are almost as good as a bath, a nice cup of tea, and a massage! (Well, maybe that's a stretch.)

Many of these warm-up exercises involve what yoga teachers call static holding. *Static holding* means you hold a position for three or more breaths. Simply stated, you push or contract a muscle against resistance and then hold that contraction for a few breaths. This technique requires a certain amount of concentration, because you have to hold the pose and focus on your breathing throughout. Static holding gives you an opportunity to stretch out your muscles and develop your ability to balance. It also gives your muscles a chance to discover new ways of moving and holding, as each exercise does its unique work for you. As you engage in static holding, listen carefully to your body, and feel your way to an understanding of which muscles you should contract and utilize fully and which muscles you should gently relax.

Chin-Chest Tuck

The purpose of the Chin-Chest Tuck is to loosen up the back of your neck and upper spine area.

Grab your hand weights and follow these steps:

1. **Stand looking straight ahead with your feet below your hips and your arms dangling at your sides, holding the weights with your palms facing inward.**

   This is the starting position. Make sure your feet are parallel to one another.

2. **Exhaling slowly, tuck your chin into your chest (see Figure 6-1); take two or three slow breaths while you're in this position.**

   If you can, touch your chin to your chest. Feel the back of your neck and upper spine stretching.

3. **Inhaling slowly, return to the starting position (see Step 1).**

Repeat this exercise three to six times, pausing to rest between each repetition.

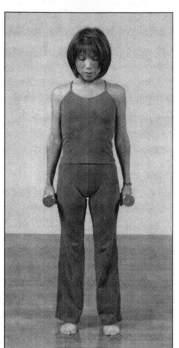

Figure 6-1:
The Chin-Chest Tuck warms up the back of your neck and your upper spine.

Head Turner

The Head Turner, as you may expect, increases the mobility of your neck, which is important for many of the yoga-with-weights exercises that require you to look in different directions.

You may want to try the Head Turner after you've been sitting at your desk for a long time to give your neck a little exercise.

Hold the hand weights as you do the Head Turner. When you're ready, follow these steps:

1. **Stand looking straight ahead with your feet below your hips and your arms dangling at your sides, holding the weights with your palms facing inward.**

   This is the starting position. Make sure your feet are parallel.

2. **Exhaling slowly and being careful not to drop your chin, turn your head and look over your right shoulder (see Figure 6-2); hold this pose for two or three slow breaths.**

   Feel the muscles of your neck contracting and stretching.

3. **Inhaling slowly, return to the starting position (see Step 1).**

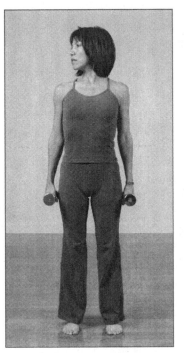

Figure 6-2:
Turning your
head and
neck is a
requirement
in many
yoga-with-
weights
exercises.

Alternating shoulders after each repetition, repeat this exercise three to six times for each shoulder.

Lateral Neck Release

The Lateral Neck Release is meant to loosen up your neck (as are the previous two warm-up exercises). We provide many neck-and-shoulder exercises because these areas are the primary places where most people carry stress. Where do you think the expression "a pain in the neck" came from?

Grab your hand weights and follow these steps:

1. **Stand looking straight ahead with your feet below your hips and your arms dangling at your sides, holding the weights with your palms facing inward.**

   This is the starting position. Make sure your feet are parallel.

2. **Exhaling slowly, lower your right ear toward your right shoulder (see Figure 6-3); hold this pose for two or three slow breaths.**

   Concentrate on the left side of your neck stretching and your left ear lifting up. Don't allow your chin to droop toward your chest. Also, concentrate on your breath opening and relaxing your neck and shoulders.

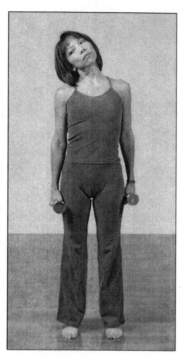

Figure 6-3:
Alleviate
your pain in
the neck
with the
Lateral
Neck
Release.

Don't stay in this position for more than three breaths; it's easy to over-stretch your neck in this position.

3. **Inhaling slowly, return your head to the starting position (see Step 1).**

Alternating sides after each repetition, repeat this exercise three to six times with each side of your neck.

Backward Shoulder Roll

The Backward Shoulder Roll loosens and relaxes the back of your shoulders and the upper back region. Time to shoulder the burden.

Pick up your hand weights and follow these steps:

1. **Stand looking straight ahead with your feet below your hips and your arms dangling at your sides, holding the weights with your palms facing inward; inhale to a count of four.**

   This is the starting position. Make sure your feet are parallel.

2. **Exhaling slowly, roll your shoulders up, back, and then down (see Figure 6-4).**

Allow the hand weights to draw your shoulders down when you lower your shoulders; the weights allow for a deeper stretch.

3. **Continue the rolling motion — moving your shoulders up, back, and then down — until they're loose as a goose.**

   Don't roll your shoulders forward; in other words, don't slouch.

Repeat this exercise three to six times.

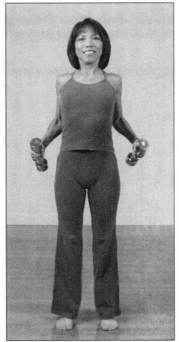

Figure 6-4:
Loosen
up your
shoulders —
no slouch-
ing allowed!

Forward Shoulder Roll

The Forward Shoulder Roll, like the Backward Shoulder Roll (see the previous exercise), loosens up and helps to relax the muscles of the front of your shoulders, your upper chest, and your back. The Forward Shoulder Roll and the Backward Shoulder Roll go hand in hand, creating a balanced workout for this area of your body.

Engage your abdominal muscles throughout this exercise to support your back.

You need hand weights for this exercise. When you're ready, follow these steps:

1. **Stand looking straight ahead with your feet below your hips and your arms dangling at your sides, holding the weights with your palms facing inward; inhale to a count of four.**

   This is the starting position. Make sure your feet are parallel.

2. **Exhaling slowly, roll your shoulders up, forward, and then down (see Figure 6-5).**

   As you roll your shoulders forward and down, allow the weights to pull your shoulders in the proper direction. Concentrate on your shoulder blades widening.

3. **Continue this motion — going up, forward, and then down — until your shoulders feel loose.**

Repeat this exercise three to six times.

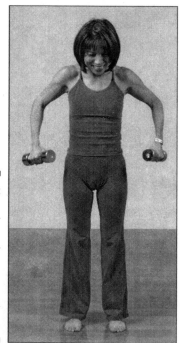

Figure 6-5:
Improve flexibility and strength in your shoulders with the Forward Shoulder Roll.

Side Bender

The Side Bender concentrates on loosening the trunk of your body — from your hips to your shoulders.

Pick up your hand weights for this exercise. When you're ready, follow these steps:

1. **Stand looking straight ahead with your feet below your hips and your arms dangling at your sides, holding the weights with your palms facing inward.**

   This is the starting position. Make sure your feet are parallel.

2. **Exhaling slowly, turn your head to the right as you lean gently to your right (see Figure 6-6); take two or three slow breaths in this position.**

   Allow the weight to stretch the left side of your body. You should feel your waistline stretching. Be careful not to lean forward or backward — lean straight to your side. Pretend you're between two walls, one in front of you and one behind.

3. **Inhaling slowly, lift your body back to the starting position (see Step 1), turning your head as you lift.**

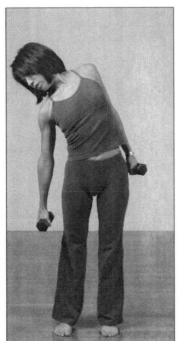

Figure 6-6:
Bend to
the side to
loosen up
the trunk of
your body.

Alternating sides after each repetition, repeat this exercise two to four times with each side of your body.

Body Twister

The Body Twister is the easiest of the warm-up exercises we provide (which is saying something, because they're all easy!). You can even try this one with a hoola-hoop if you're so inclined. The object of the exercise is to loosen your hips and improve the flexibility of your trunk as a whole.

You need hand weights for this exercise. When you're ready, follow these steps:

1. **Stand looking straight ahead with your feet below your hips and the weights held at hip level, palms facing inward.**

   This is the starting position. Make sure your feet are parallel.

2. **Pressing down on your left foot, twist your trunk, neck, head, and shoulders to the right (see Figure 6-7). Hold this pose for two or three relaxed breaths.**

3. **Return your upper half to the starting position (see Step 1) and take the pressure off your left foot.**

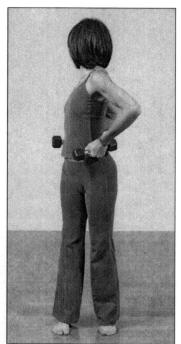

Figure 6-7:
A warm-up exercise with a twist!

Alternating from side to side, repeat this exercise six to eight times on each side of your body.

Wrist Rotator

The Wrist Rotator loosens and relaxes your wrists, a must for the times when you have to maneuver hand weights or support your body with your hands.

You need hand weights for this exercise. If you have carpal tunnel syndrome or another wrist condition, however, use light hand weights to prevent injury or no hand weights at all.

When you have your hand weights ready, follow these steps:

1. **Stand looking straight ahead with your feet below your hips and your arms dangling at your sides, holding the weights with your palms facing backward.**

   This is the starting position. Make sure your feet are parallel.

2. **Breathing slowly and steadily, rotate your wrists in a counter-clockwise fashion until the backs of your hands are facing each other (see Figure 6-8).**

   Enjoy feeling the muscles of your wrists loosen.

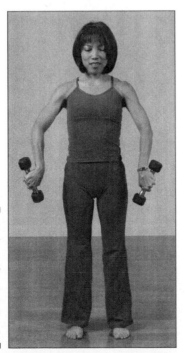

Figure 6-8:
Give your wrists a workout by rotating them with hand weights.

3. **Continuing to breathe slowly and steadily, rotate your wrists in the clockwise direction until your palms are facing forward.**

Repeat this exercise three to six times in each direction.

Big Shoulder Release

The Big Shoulder Release is designed to eliminate the tension in your shoulders, shoulder joints, and upper back.

Grab your hand weights for this exercise and follow these steps:

1. **Stand looking straight ahead with your shoulders squared, your feet directly below your hips, and your arms hanging to your sides, holding the weights with your palms facing backward.**

   This is the starting position. Press down onto all four corners of your feet, and draw your belly in and up to support your back. Make sure your feet are parallel.

2. **Inhaling to a count of four, raise your arms forward and up, following the weights with your eyes as you lift (see Figure 6-9).**

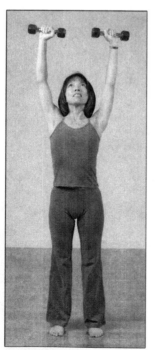

Figure 6-9:
You have to eliminate the tension in your shoulders to do yoga with weights effectively.

Lift, don't throw, your arms so they're straight over your shoulders, and hold them there for a moment.

Don't jerk your arms, overextend the weights, or slouch. Performing these actions with weights in your hands can cause muscle or joint injury.

3. **Exhaling to a count of four, lower your arms and head to the starting position (see Step 1).**

Repeat this exercise three or four times.

Y Shoulder Release

The Y Shoulder Release is designed to strengthen and improve the flexibility of your shoulders and upper back.

You need hand weights for this exercise. When you're ready, follow these steps:

1. **With your shoulders squared and feet below your hips, stand looking straight ahead with your arms hanging to your sides, holding the weights with your palms facing inward.**

   This is the starting position. Press onto all four corners of your feet, and draw your belly in and up to support your back.

2. **Inhaling to a count of four, raise your arms away from your sides until they form a Y with your body, looking toward the ceiling as you lift (see Figure 6-10).**

   Be careful not to jerk your arms, which can cause muscle or joint injury.

   If you can't lift your arms above your shoulders, lift them as high as you comfortably can.

3. **Exhaling to a count of four, lower your arms and gaze to the starting position (see Step 1).**

Repeat this exercise three or four times.

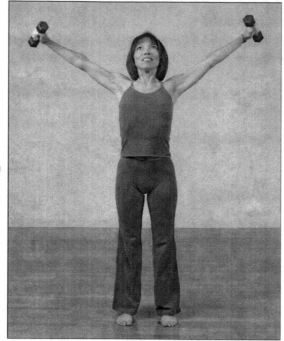

Figure 6-10:
Warming up and strengthening your shoulders also benefits your back and chest.

Quad Stretcher

The Quad Stretcher warms up your quads (or quadriceps), the large muscles on the front of your legs above your knees, by stretching them and strengthening them with the help of ankle weights.

You need ankle weights and a chair for balance in this exercise. When you're ready, follow these steps:

1. **Stand behind the back of the chair with your feet directly below your hips and your arms at your sides.**

   This is the starting position.

2. **Bend your right knee, reach back with your right hand to hold your foot, and hold the chair with your left hand for balance (see Figure 6-11); hold this position for three or four deep, full breaths.**

   Make sure your shoulders are over your hips and your knees are close to one another. Feel your quad muscle stretching.

   If you can't reach your foot, grab a pant leg. You can also put a towel around your ankle and hold the towel.

3. **Return to the starting position (see Step 1).**

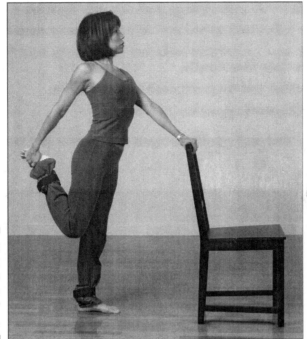

Figure 6-11:
Make like a
crane as
you warm
up your
quads.

Alternating legs after each repetition, repeat this exercise four to six times with each leg.

Back and Hamstring Stretcher

The Back and Hamstring Stretcher works your hamstrings and, in the process, stretches and strengthens your back. Your hamstring is the long muscle on the back of your leg that runs from your knee to your buttock. To stretch two areas with one stone, read on!

You need a chair and your ankle weights for this exercise. When you're ready, follow these steps:

1. **Stand behind the back of a chair with your feet directly below your hips and your arms at your sides.**

2. **Grab the back of the chair with both hands and step backward by one arm's length, making sure your arms and the trunk of your body are parallel with the floor.**

   This is the starting position. Fix your gaze on the floor.

3. **Step forward with your right leg, and flex your right foot.**

   Draw your belly in and up and your tailbone down for support.

4. **Lean back onto both of your heels (see Figure 6-12); hold this position for three or four slow breaths.**

   Concentrate on your hamstrings and back stretching.

5. **Return to the starting position (see Step 2).**

Alternating legs after each repetition, repeat this exercise four to six times with each leg.

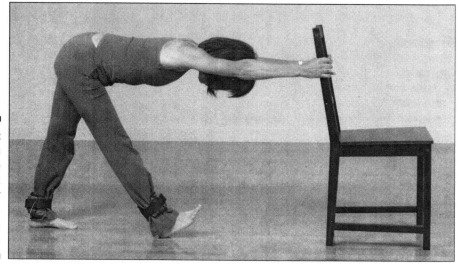

Figure 6-12:
You can warm up your back and your legs with one warm-up exercise.

All-Out Hamstring Stretcher

Your hamstring is a long muscle located on the backside of your leg. It extends from your buttock to the back of your knee. The All-Out Hamstring Stretcher stretches your hamstrings — an important task because these muscles help you move comfortably in many of the exercises where you need to step, stand, or bend over.

Grab a chair and strap on your ankle weights. When you're ready, follow these steps:

1. **Face the front of the chair with your feet below your hips and your hands on your thighs.**

   This is the starting position.

2. **Put your right heel on the chair's seat.**

   Keep your foot flexed and your toes pointing toward the ceiling. Pull your belly in and up and draw your tailbone down to anchor your legs.

3. **Bend forward as far as you can to stretch your hamstring, keeping both legs as straight as possible (see Figure 6-13); hold this pose for three or four slow breaths.**

   If you can, put both of your hands on the chair (see Figure 6-13). You should also feel your back stretching.

4. **Return to the starting position (see Step 1) by slowly raising your body and taking your right heel off the chair.**

Alternating legs after each repetition, repeat this exercise four to six times with each leg.

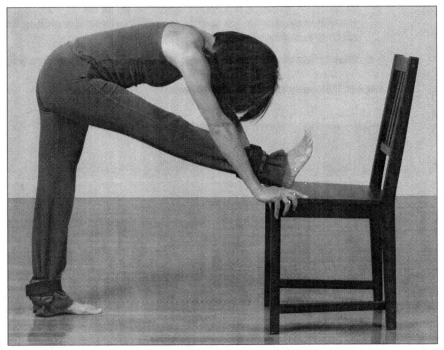

Figure 6-13:
A classic hamstring stretch.

The Big Stretcher

The Big Stretcher warms up your shoulders, back, and spine. The pose may seem difficult at first if you aren't limber, but the discomfort is worth it because the exercise stretches many different muscles that help you in yoga-with-weights workouts.

Strap on your ankle weights and follow these steps:

1. **Stand with your shoulders squared, your feet below your hips, and your arms hanging to your sides.**

2. **Interlace your fingers behind your back, with your palms facing each other.**

   This is the starting position. You may have to raise your shoulders — in other words, shrug them — to do this.

   If you can't interlace your fingers, grab a hand towel behind your back with both hands.

3. **As you slowly exhale, bend your knees and move the trunk of your body forward as far as you can (see Figure 6-14); hold this pose for three or four breaths.**

   If you can go forward until you're looking at your feet like the model in Figure 6-14, great. If not, don't worry — go as far as you can. Your arms should remain together and be pointing toward the ceiling. Press onto all four corners of each foot.

4. **Slowly inhale as you return to the starting position (see Step 2).**

Repeat this exercise six to eight times.

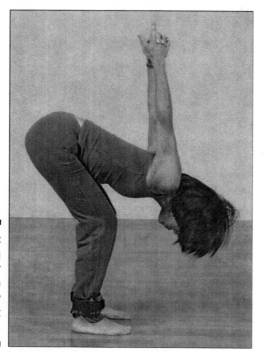

Figure 6-14:
The Big
Stretcher
warms up
many
different
muscles.

Marching Legs

In the Marching Legs warm-up exercise, you get to pretend that you're in a marching band. This exercise warms up your hips and gluts (the muscles on your buttocks).

If you want to go for a jog or do some other aerobic activity in place of yoga with weights, Marching Legs is an excellent warm-up for running activities.

You need both ankle weights and hand weights for this exercise. When you're ready, follow these steps:

1. **Stand looking straight ahead with your feet below your hips and your arms hanging to your sides, holding the hand weights with your palms facing inward.**

   This is the starting position. Make sure your feet are parallel and that your shoulders are squared.

2. **As you slowly inhale to a count of four, lift your right knee (see Figure 6-15).**

   Pull your belly in for support, and keep your shoulders squared.

3. **As you slowly exhale to a count of four, lower your right leg to the starting position (see Step 1).**

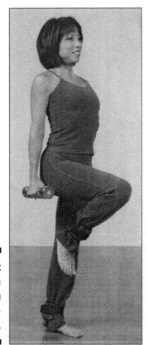

Figure 6-15:
Start a parade with this warm-up exercise.

Alternating legs after each repetition, repeat this exercise six to eight times with each leg.

Hip Opener

The Hip Opener is an excellent stretch for your buttocks and hamstrings. It provides freedom and a greater range of motion in those areas, which in turn supports the well-being and healthy movement of your hips.

Keep your belly muscles engaged at all times during this exercise.

You need ankle weights for this exercise. When you're ready, follow these steps:

1. **Lay on the floor with your knees bent and your feet flat on the floor.**

2. **Place your right ankle on the top of your left knee (see Figure 6-16a).**

   This is the starting position.

3. **Draw your left knee toward your chest (see Figure 6-16b); hold this pose for two or three long, slow breaths.**

   Hold the underside of your left thigh with both hands to help bring your thigh closer to your chest. Pull your belly in for support.

4. **Slowly lower your left foot back to the floor and put your right leg back in the starting position (see Figure 6-16a).**

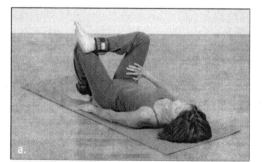

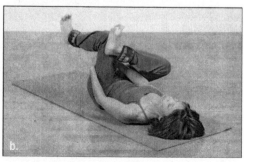

Figure 6-16: Stretch out your entire lower body, from the hips to the feet.

Alternating legs after each repetition, repeat this exercise six to eight times with each leg.

Lower Back Release

The object of the Lower Back Release is to gently stretch your lower back, hips, and pelvis and to relieve tension in these areas.

For a better stretch, keep your buttocks on the floor throughout this exercise.

You need ankle weights for this exercise. When you're ready, follow these steps:

1. **Lay on your back with your knees bent and your heels a few inches away from your buttocks (see Figure 6-17a).**

   This is the starting position.

2. **Slowly inhaling to a count of four, lift the lumbar curve of your back toward the ceiling (see Figure 6-17b).**

   The *lumbar curve* of your back is the part of your back between your waist and the base of your spine. Let your back rise to the rhythm of your breathing. Pull your belly in and up for support, and tilt your tailbone and pubic bone toward your navel.

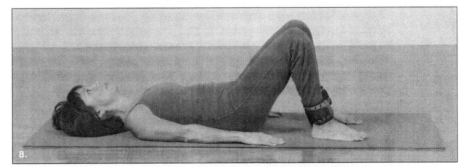

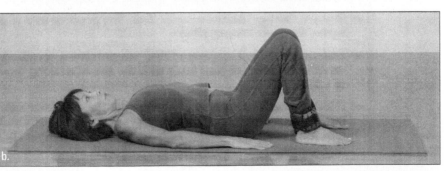

Figure 6-17: Your lower back supports you during many yoga-with-weights exercises.

3. **Slowly exhaling to a count of four, lower your back to the starting position (see Figure 6-17a).**

   Let your back fall to the rhythm of your breathing.

Repeat this exercise six to eight times.

Knowing the Benefits of Meditation

When many people hear the word "meditate," they think of a man in a loin-cloth with a serene look on his face sitting cross-legged on top of a mountain. Meditation, however, isn't nearly as esoteric as people think. It doesn't require years of study or mystical knowledge from on high; all it takes is practice.

Meditation is a spontaneous flow of consciousness when all the conditions are just right. It's about listening inwardly with a quiet mind for the wisdom and guidance of a more expansive and unlimited mind.

All the arts of relaxation — breath control, contemplation, prayer, affirmation, repetition of a mantra, and visualization — are different, but they all direct you toward self-realization and a deep meditative state. Different systems of thought and traditions vary in their meditation techniques, but they all have the same goal: to reach the point of stillness, quiet, and communion with the essence of your being.

With meditation, you discover how to quiet your mind and increase your level of energy and enjoyment of life. You experience the natural joy of being in meditation, and you establish a greater confidence and a higher understanding. Meditation can deliver deep inner peace; increase your mental stamina; improve your memory; enlarge your multitasking abilities; and teach you to organize your internal awareness and concentration.

You can practice different forms of meditation:

- **Mantra meditation:** You focus your attention on a repeated word, thought, or sound.

- **Metta or loving kindness meditation:** You practice acts of generosity or loving kindness toward others.

- **Stair-step meditation (or modified progressive relaxation):** You focus on different areas of your body with the aim of relaxing those areas one at a time.

- **Mindfulness:** You observe whatever goes through your mind without judging or analyzing it. (Some yoga practitioners don't consider this a true form of meditation, but rather a practice or deeper step toward meditation.)

Meditation as a garden

Here's one useful way to consider meditation: Imagine your mind as a garden. In a garden, you want only the plants that you plant yourself — vegetables, flowers, and fruit trees — to grow, but at every opportunity, weeds spring up to choke off your plants. Those weeds are like the chatter that goes on in most people's heads most of the time. Consider all the urgent thoughts, distractions, and mind-chatter that go through your head in a single day. The average person thinks 60,000 thoughts each day, and as much as 80 percent of these thoughts are repetitive. You thought them yesterday, and unless you begin to change your thought habits, you'll think them again tomorrow and the day after

that. Unless you train your mind, this chatter will go on year after year.

Meditation practice is how you train your mind. It can quiet or silence some of your thoughts in order to keep the weeds from growing out of control. Meditation is a way to nurture the plants in the garden that you want to grow by bringing you into the present and letting you focus on your inner domain. As a gardener cultivates a garden, meditation cultivates the essential things inside you that really matter. The goal of meditation is to *be* in the moment as it unfolds and connect to the state, or fruit, of your being.

Cooling Down: Ending Your Workout with Meditation

In each of the workout chapters in this book, we ask you to meditate whenever you complete a yoga-with-weights workout. Meditation is an excellent way to cool down after you exercise. It rests your body and mind, and it serves as a soothing and supportive transition between your workout and the next activity you want to engage in. This section introduces some useful meditation techniques and the proper way to end your meditation session so you can move on with your day.

If you want to explore meditation further, we recommend *Yoga For Dummies,* by Georg Feuerstein and Larry Payne (Wiley), and *Meditation For Dummies,* by Stephan Bodian and Dean Ornish (Wiley).

Looking at some meditation techniques

We advise you to meditate after each yoga-with-weights workout in all our workout chapters, but we also encourage you to meditate whenever the mood strikes you. The more you practice meditating, the easier it is to sit still without getting distracted or letting your mind wander. Be patient with yourself as you practice. Practice and more practice will help.

How long you meditate is up to you. You can use an alarm to make a sound after a certain amount of time elapses, or you can purchase gentle chiming timers designed for meditation practice that chime softly so as not to startle you (Brookstone, Whole Foods, Sharper Image, and other stores sell them). Start by meditating for a few minutes and build up to 20, 45, or even 60 minutes over time. Try to meditate three times a week at minimum, and meditate daily if you can. At first, your mind will wander, but eventually you'll be able to maintain your focus as you move into deeper states of meditation. Be patient, and meditate without any expectations.

Following are some meditation techniques you can use on your own time or after yoga-with-weights workouts.

Sit in silence

Sit comfortably in a cross-legged position on the floor (and preferably on your yoga mat).

If sitting on the floor isn't easy for you, put a small, firm cushion or folded blanket under your buttocks, or sit on the edge of a wooden chair with your feet on the floor (don't sit on an upholstered chair, because they tend to induce drowsiness). You can also lie down or sit against a wall.

Rest your hands on your knees with your palms up or down. Sit with your spine straight, and remain silent, concentrating on the world around you. This will heighten your awareness and allow you to focus on your breathing.

Focus on your breath

You can use your breath as a tool to calm your active mind and direct your consciousness into new and deeper levels of awareness and insight.

Let your breath flow smoothly, evenly, and consistently, with the air moving in and out of your lungs like waves on a seashore. Breathe soundlessly or near soundlessly through your nostrils. Notice your lungs expanding as you inhale, and relaxing as you exhale. Breathe from your navel to your heart and into your chest, upper back, and shoulders. Without forcing, let the breath penetrate into the deepest recesses of your lungs.

Relax systematically

Go into a deep meditation by taking inventory of the different parts of your body. As you breathe in and out, concentrate on relaxing, beginning with your forehead and scalp and then moving to your eyes, cheeks, ears, the corners of your mouth, your tongue, your teeth, and the hinges of your jaw. Feel your breath moving throughout your body, and let the tensions dissolve.

Relax in your throat, neck, and shoulders. Take a soft and gentle breath into your right nostril and relax the right side of your body. Now do the same with your left nostril and the left side of your body. You can then breathe through both nostrils and invite the breath to move down into your pelvis and hips to relax them. Imagine that you're breathing into your left leg, and then do the same with your right leg. Imagine that the air you're breathing is flowing straight into each leg. As you breathe out, relax fully.

Scan your body to deepen stillness and release tension

For three to ten breaths, scan your entire body as you breathe. Feel your body breathing all at once from the inside out. Without forcing, breathe in so completely, yet gently, that you feel your breath moving into the outermost edges of your body and even to areas beyond where your eyes can see. If you still feel any sensations of constriction in your body, contract and squeeze the muscles in the constricted areas of your body. For example, if your hip or thigh feels constricted, contract the muscles that surround those areas, squeezing and releasing the muscles. This helps to increase blood circulation to the areas that feel constricted.

Use word repetition

Repeating words gives your mind the power to stay focused on the task at hand. It moves you deeper into a meditative state.

Choose a positive-affirmation word that works for you — you may want to choose *peace, harmony,* or *well-being,* for example. Silently, hearing only the inner voice of your mind, repeat the word internally again and again as you breathe in and out. Feel your brain embracing the positive influence, vibration, and nature of the word.

Meditate with the use of sound

Sit still and listen to the sounds around you without thinking about where the sounds originated or what the sounds mean. Just hear them. Ideally, you should be outside and listening to the sounds of nature — the wind, birds, the rustle of leaves. Obviously, no cell phones or other electronic distractions are allowed in this type of meditation. We don't recommend listening to music during meditation because, well, that's listening to music, not meditating.

Moving into silence

Become your own observer. Notice your thoughts, step back from them, and watch them with your mind as they appear and pass by. Meanwhile, feel the breath moving throughout your body and let any tensions dissolve breath by breath, moment into moment, into nothingness. Let this meditation be a simple yet profound path toward your discovery of what's real and meaningful in your life.

Ending your meditation

To end your meditation session, follow these steps:

1. **In a sitting position, open your eyes gently.**

2. **Take a deep breath and close your eyes again.**

3. **Open your eyes and feel the peaceful sense of calm and awareness.**

4. **Place your hands on the top of your chest, in the upper chest and collarbone area.**

5. **Inhale through your nose and, with your lips slightly pursed, breathe out through your mouth, making a gentle whooshing sound.**

6. **Take three more deep-cleansing breaths with your eyes open.**

   Feel the sensations of your physical body as you sit there.

7. **Take your time before rising to pause for a moment and take stock of how refreshed, confident, and sure you feel.**

Chapter 7

From Head to Toe: The Balanced Workout

In This Chapter

▶ Loosening your entire body

▶ Releasing tension from muscles, head to toe

▶ Breathing consciously and mindfully as you strengthen your core

▶ Relaxing your body for the rest of your day

*W*e designed the Balanced Workout in this chapter to exercise and tone your entire body in one workout session. In this workout, you exercise all the major muscle groups of your body, from head to toe. The exercises strengthen your bones, maintain joint flexibility, lengthen muscles, and release tension held in tight muscles — all while you become perfectly aware and perfectly relaxed. If you do these exercises on a regular basis, you'll take a giant step toward the goal of getting in shape and cultivating a calm mind and beautiful body.

The Balanced Workout takes 20 to 30 minutes. Ideally, you should practice it every other day. Of course, staying fit and finding the time for exercise can be a challenge, but we urge you to take the time to do this workout. You'll notice your health improving in a matter of days — it's what we call personal transformation, and the potential is unlimited. (For reasons why yoga with weights is a timesaver, turn to Chapter 3, and for motivational tips, turn to Chapter 19.)

If you're new to yoga with weights, you may wonder why you have to pay so much attention to breathing. In every exercise, we tell you when to inhale and exhale and how long to inhale and exhale, and between exercises, we instruct you to pause for deep and steady breaths. We have you focus on breathing because breathing correctly helps you to feel emotionally centered, physically stronger, and mentally alert. In the Balanced Workout, you use the Complete

Breath, which fills your body from your chest to your belly (Chapter 4 explains what the Complete Breath is). Breathing Complete Breaths is a mindful practice that harmonizes body, mind, and spirit; improves your circulation; and de-stresses your mind.

The Mountain

The Mountain is based on a traditional yoga master pose (meaning it affects every system in your body). It's a warm-up exercise that loosens and relaxes your spine, shoulders, and neck. It opens up your chest, back, and spine for vitality, and for these reasons, it's good for your posture. The exercise also establishes a foundation so you can focus on concentration and is wonderful for developing balance and coordination.

Grab your hand weights before you climb the Mountain. When you're ready to go, follow these steps:

1. **Stand with your legs as far apart as your hips and your toes pointing straight ahead, and let the hand weights dangle at your sides with your palms facing backward (see Figure 7-1a).**

   This is the starting position. Look straight ahead with your chin neither lifted nor lowered.

2. **As you inhale to a count of four, step forward with your right leg and lift the weights above your shoulders (see Figure 7-1b).**

   Keep your arms straight and raise them directly above your shoulders. Draw your belly in and up and your tailbone down for support. Focus on how you distribute your body weight as you step forward.

   If you feel any pinching in your shoulders or neck, you can lift the weights halfway up, perpendicular to your body.

   As you lift, the heel of your back foot may leave the floor, but keep the ball of your foot planted (see Figure 7-1b). Concentrate on your breathing and alignment during the lift. Make sure your breathing is steady and even. Don't shrug your shoulders.

3. **As you exhale to a count of four, lower your arms and step back into the starting position (see Figure 7-1a).**

   Lower the weight in time to your breathing. Don't look up or look down — gaze straight ahead.

Alternating legs, repeat this exercise six to eight times with each leg. Pause to rest, and then do six to eight more repetitions with each leg.

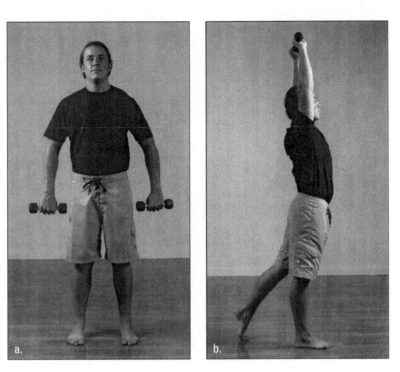

Figure 7-1:
The Mountain is a head-to-toe exercise that loosens your body.

Heaven and Earth

This exercise is called Heaven and Earth because you reach to the sky and root to the earth at the same time. It stretches the side of your body and brings oxygen to your back and spine; it helps you warm up and focus on your breathing; and it gets the energy flowing through your body.

Grab your hand weights and follow these steps to reach for the heavens:

1. **Stand with your legs as far apart as your hips and your toes pointing straight ahead, and let the hand weights dangle at your sides with your palms facing inward (see Figure 7-2a).**

   This is the starting position.

2. **Inhaling to a count to four, extend the weight in your right hand forward and then above your right shoulder, following the weight with your eyes (see Figure 7-2b).**

   Stretch out your arm and shoulder as much as possible without lifting your heels off the ground, and press your right foot into the ground as you look to the sky. You should finish inhaling as the weight reaches its peak. Feel your hip and the side of your body stretch as you lift the weight.

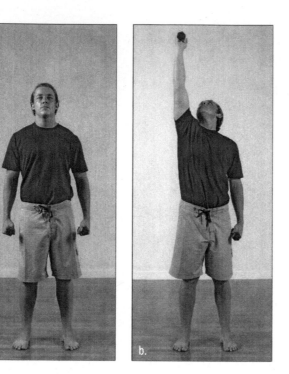

Figure 7-2:
Heaven
and Earth
invigorates
your body
and helps
you breathe.

If your neck feels too tight, look toward your elbow; in other words, look as high as you comfortably can. If your shoulders are tight, practice this exercise without a weight or raise the weight halfway.

3. **Exhaling to a count of four, lower the weight back to your side and return to the starting position (see Figure 7-2a).**

Keep your feet squarely on the floor throughout this exercise. Don't throw the weight — gently lift it. Focus on your breathing so that you have smooth transitions as you inhale (when you lift the weight) and exhale (when you lower the weight). Try to time your breathing so that you never hold your breath. Your breathing helps you relax and do the stretching portion of this exercise.

Repeat this exercise six to eight times with each arm, pause to rest, and then do six to eight more repetitions with each arm.

The Rag Doll

The Rag Doll releases tension in the parts of your body where most people carry tension — your neck and spine. It helps you relax and also works your abdominal muscles and the core muscles of your torso for a total upper-body workout.

Pick up your hand weights and follow these steps:

1. **Standing with your feet directly below your hips and your toes pointing forward, let your hand weights dangle at your sides with your palms facing inward (see Figure 7-3a).**

   This is the starting position. Don't let your belly collapse in this exercise — sculpt your belly in and up. Let your abdominal muscles support your spine. You should feel an "energetic girdle" around your abdomen.

   Throughout this exercise, keep your feet parallel to one another, both pointing straight ahead. Don't turn them out.

2. **Inhaling to a count of four, slowly roll your shoulders up and forward (see Figure 7-3b).**

   Pause your breath momentarily when you reach the top of the shoulder roll.

3. **Exhaling to a count of four, bend your knees and roll your torso forward with your shoulders leading the way (see Figure 7-3c).**

   Now you're in the rag doll position, with your neck, head, and shoulders feeling loose and relaxed. Don't shrug your shoulders — roll them forward, using the weights to help extend your body forward and lengthen your spine.

   You should feel your spine stretching as the weights hang. Keep your knees slightly bent and move your hips back.

4. **Inhaling to a count of four and pressing through your legs, roll your shoulders up, back, and down as you return to the starting position (see Figure 7-3a).**

   Feel the breath filling your lungs during this part of the exercise.

5. **Exhale to a count of four as you rest in the starting position.**

Do this exercise six to eight times, pause to rest, and then repeat the exercise another six to eight times.

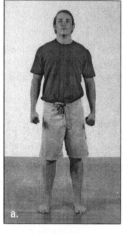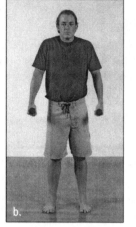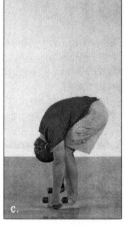

Figure 7-3:
The Rag Doll releases tension in your neck and spine and improves your flexibility and mobility.

The Airplane

The Airplane raises the altitude of your attitude, making you feel uplifted. It stimulates feel-good chemistry in your brain and works your biceps, triceps, and upper torso. Imagine that you're flying through blue skies as you do this exercise.

You need the hand weights for this exercise; ankle weights are optional. Use the ankle weights if you want additional tone and strength. Adding the extra weight exercises your legs a bit more.

Follow these steps to fly the Airplane:

1. **Stand with your feet together and directly below your hips, and hold the weights in front of your chest with the knuckles of each hand touching (see Figure 7-4a).**

   This is the starting position.

2. **Slowly inhaling to a count of four, bend your left knee, extend your right leg behind you as you lean forward, and open your arms to a C position (see Figure 7-4b).**

   While you're extending your leg, look slightly upward toward your forehead and brow. To achieve the C position, imagine you're crunching a soda can with your shoulder blades.

   To help with balancing, press your standing foot into the floor, draw your belly in and up, and draw your tailbone down.

If you feel pinched in your neck and shoulders or you otherwise experience distress as you maneuver the hand weights, use lighter weights or no weights at all.

3. **Slowly exhaling to a count of four, return the hand weights to your chest as you lower your leg to the floor and assume the starting position (see Figure 7-4a).**

Repeat this exercise six to eight times with each leg, pause to rest, and then do the exercise six to eight more times with each leg.

Figure 7-4:
In the Airplane, you work your balancing muscles and strengthen your upper body.

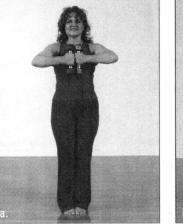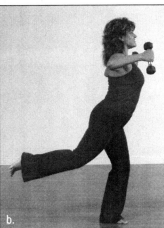

The Triangle

The Triangle is based on a powerful and ancient yoga master pose. It's an extended side angle pose that beginners can enjoy. The exercise works many muscles in your body, but it concentrates on the core muscles of your trunk, your shoulders, and your legs. As you balance, the Triangle also helps you trace and explore the physical feeling and sensation of your body.

You need hand weights for this exercise, so grab them and follow these steps:

1. **With your feet parallel to each other, stand with your legs as wide apart as you comfortably can, and hold the weights at your waist with your palms facing inward.**

2. **Turn both feet to the right and bend at the right knee until you align your knee over your ankle (see Figure 7-5a).**

3. **Rotate your torso to the right and rest your right forearm on your right thigh or knee; let the weight in your left hand hang to the ground with your arm straight and your palm facing inward (see Figure 7-5b).**

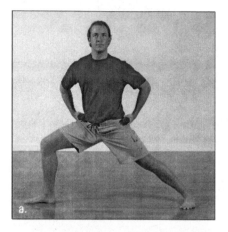
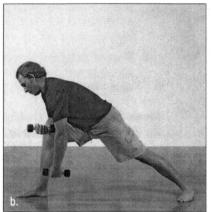
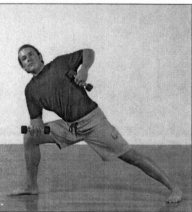

Figure 7-5:
The Triangle
is a yoga
master pose
(with a few
variations)
that
beginners
can master.

This is the starting position.

REMEMBER

Draw your belly in and up and your tailbone down to stabilize your legs, trunk, and spine. If you feel a burning sensation along the top of your supporting leg, your leg is doing too much support work. Focus on the core muscles of your torso and trunk so that they do more of the lifting and balancing work.

4. **Exhaling to a count of four, lift the weight in your left hand to your torso, bending your elbow toward the ceiling and drawing your shoulder slightly back, over, and downward as you lift (see Figure 7-5c).**

   Look toward the ceiling and imagine that you're pulling back an arrow on a bow. You should feel a solid pulling action that goes up, over, and back with each lift.

5. **Inhaling to a count of four, bring your head and torso back down as you turn to the right and lower the weight to the starting position (see Figure 7-5b).**

Follow the weight with your eyes. Don't drop the weight — lower it slowly to the floor.

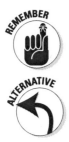

To anchor yourself, press down onto all four corners of your right foot and onto the balls of your left foot as you do this exercise. Don't let your supporting knee wobble from side to side or extend over your toes.

If you're flexible enough, straighten both legs as you do this exercise. If you feel a strain in your neck, use lighter weights.

Do this exercise six to eight times on each leg, pause to rest, and then do the exercise six to eight more times on each leg.

The Exalted Warrior

The Exalted Warrior makes use of a classic yoga pose — the victorious warrior. You feel the strength, honor, and courage of a warrior as you do this exercise; it sends a surge of power through your entire body. It strengthens and tones your upper torso, opens your collarbone, teaches you to work the core muscles of your trunk for balance, and strengthens your legs.

Pick up your hand weights for this exercise and follow these steps:

1. **Stand with your feet together and your toes pointing forward, and allow the hand weights to dangle at your sides with your palms facing backward.**

2. **Gently step back with your right foot, keeping your legs straight.**

   Turn your back foot slightly out for balance and stability. Align your shoulders with your hips.

   Make sure your legs are strong and engaged. Let your back and your front leg support you.

3. **Raise your arms forward until they're directly above your shoulders (see Figure 7-6a).**

   This is the starting position. Draw your belly in and up and point your tailbone down throughout the rest of the exercise.

4. **As you exhale to a count of four, pull your arms down, bending your elbows and holding the weights at ear-level (see Figure 7-6b).**

   This movement is what weightlifters call a *back-lat pull-down*. Pull down with your *lats* — the muscles on your back around your shoulder blades — as well as with your shoulders. Don't let your wrists flop or cock back as you do this exercise; keep them aligned with your forearms.

5. **As you inhale to a count of four, press the weights back up to the starting position (see Figure 7-6a).**

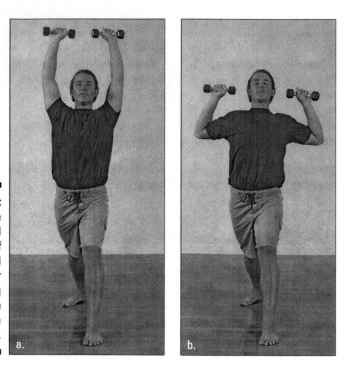

Do this exercise six to eight times on each leg, pause to rest, and then do the exercise six to eight more times on each leg.

The Warrior II

The Warrior II is a variation of the Exalted Warrior, the previous exercise in this workout. This version works your biceps, legs, and the core muscles of your trunk and torso. It looks easy, but if you do it right, the exercise works your entire body and teaches you the power of concentration.

Pick up your hand weights for this exercise and follow these steps:

1. **Stand with your legs as far apart as you comfortably can and your feet pointing forward, and hold the weights at your waist with your palms facing forward.**

2. **Turn both of your feet to the right and bend your right knee until you align it vertically with your ankle.**

   Your back foot should be pointing at a 45-degree angle, and your right foot should be pointing straight ahead to your right. Keep your torso centered equally between your heels and your hips rotated wide open. You're in a lunge position.

3. **Raise your arms to shoulder height with your palms facing upward and your arms extended away from your body (see Figure 7-7a).**

   This is the starting position. Concentrate on your legs to keep them strong and stable as you move your arms.

4. **Exhaling to a count of four, draw your hands to your shoulders with a bicep curl (see Figure 7-7b).**

   Draw your belly in and up and your tailbone down to support yourself and maintain your balance. The Warrior II is a total body exercise, not just a biceps exercise. Don't let your front knee wobble or move forward over your toes.

5. **Inhaling to a count of four, return to the starting position (see Figure 7-7a).**

Do this exercise six to eight times on each leg, pause to rest, and then do six to eight more repetitions on each leg.

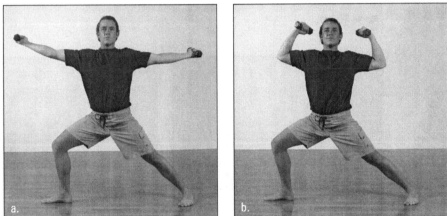

Figure 7-7:
Flex your arm muscles and maintain balance with your legs as you do the Warrior II.

The Camel

Tired of leaning forward all day to look at your computer screen or lift boxes off the ground? If so, the Camel — a classic yoga pose — is for you. It's a simple exercise, but it has real benefits. It stretches out your spine; tones your thighs and backside; opens up your chest, armpits, and back; and improves circulation to your lungs and heart region. In most daily activities, you lean forward, but this exercise gives you an opportunity to stretch the other direction.

If you have sensitive knees, don't sit on your heels during this exercise. Try straddling a rolled-up yoga mat, a stack of books, or a briefcase.

Grab your hand weights for this exercise and follow these steps:

1. **Sit on your knees with your buttocks resting on your heels and your legs flat on the floor, and hold the weights at your sides with your palms facing backward (see Figure 7-8a).**

   This is the starting position. Look straight ahead, and keep your spine erect.

2. **As you inhale to a count of four, rise to your knees — using the power and strength of your thigh muscles — and lift the weights straight above your shoulders (see Figure 7-8b).**

   Let your breath establish a rhythm as you rise and lift.

3. **As you exhale to a count of four, sit down on your legs, and lower the weights to the starting position (see Figure 7-8a).**

   Don't swing the weights. Carefully control the release as you kneel and sit back down.

Do this exercise six to eight times, pause to rest, and then do it six to eight more times.

Figure 7-8:
Focus on your breathing as you lift your body off the ground.

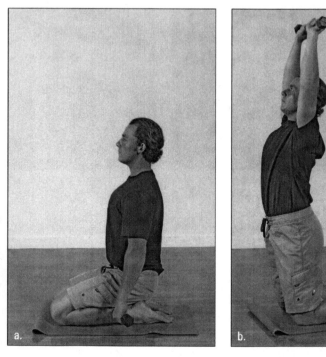

The Table

Remember your mom telling you to sit up straight at the dinner table? Well, she would approve of this exercise, called the Table. It works and tones your buttocks, hips, and thighs; it exercises your back and spine to develop core-strength conditioning; and it helps you develop the muscles that support your trunk. Overall, this exercise helps you develop good posture. You also kick like a donkey and develop leg strength, which your mom probably didn't approve of at the table.

Time to grab your ankle weights. After you're strapped in, follow these steps:

1. **Get on all fours with your hands directly below your shoulders and your knees directly under your hips.**

   Lift your waistline so that your back feels flat. Spread your fingers wide so they support your weight.

2. **Lift your right leg up to the height of your hip, keeping the plane of your body flat (see Figure 7-9a).**

   This is the starting position.

3. **Inhaling to a count of four, bend your knee backward and push your leg up (see Figure 7-9b).**

   Press your foot up so it's higher than your hip, without rolling your hip to the side. Keep your leg directly behind you and your hips squared. Flex your foot as if you're standing on the floor.

   If you feel discomfort in your lower back, don't raise your leg as high. Use a lighter weight if you have trouble lifting your leg.

4. **Exhaling to a count of four, unbend your knee and bring your leg back to the starting position (see Figure 7-9a).**

Let your breathing guide you. Slowly move your foot upward as you inhale; move it back down slowly as you exhale. Count to four as you complete each inhale and exhale.

Don't push with your arms or bend your elbows. Use them only for stability and maintaining your balance. Don't sag as you do this exercise.

Do this exercise six to eight times with each leg, pause to rest, and then do it six to eight more times with each leg.

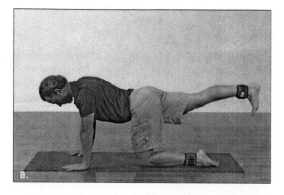

Figure 7-9:
The Table
encourages
good
posture at
the dinner
table and
elsewhere.

The Cat

Cats are experts when it comes to stretching, so it should come as no surprise that the Cat stretches out your spine, back, neck, and shoulders. This exercise works the same muscles as the Table (see the previous exercise in this workout), but you also stretch your spine and belly. Take your inspiration from a cat as you work through this exercise; do it a few times, and you'll be good at stretching, too.

You need to strap on your ankle weights for this exercise. Ready to go? Follow these steps:

1. **Get on all fours with your knees directly under your hips and your hands directly below your shoulders.**

   Make sure your fingers are spread wide for support.

2. **Extend your right leg behind you, and look forward and up (see Figure 7-10a).**

   This is the starting position. Draw your belly in and up and your tailbone down for support.

Don't rotate your leg (what a dog does next to a fire hydrant). Make sure it's in line with the rest of your body.

3. **Exhaling to a count of four, draw your right leg deep into your chest as you arch your back and look toward your navel (see Figure 7-10b).**

   Point your nose at your pelvis as you move toward your bent knee. Don't swing your leg; move it slowly in rhythm with your breathing.

4. **Breathe four counts in and four counts out while in the tucked position.**

5. **Inhaling to a count of four, lift your head, flatten your back, and extend your right leg back to the starting position (see Figure 7-10a).**

Keep your arms straight to stabilize and balance your body throughout this exercise. Make sure they stay directly below your shoulders.

Do this exercise six to eight times with each leg, pause to rest, and then do it six to eight more times with each leg.

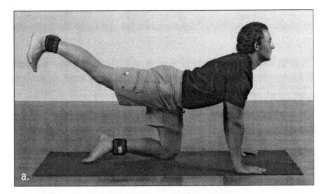

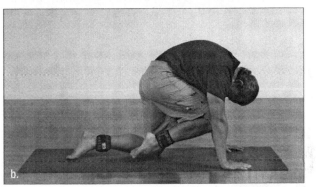

Figure 7-10:
Stretch your
back like a
cat in this
exercise.

The Dog

The Dog introduces ankle weights to a classic yoga master pose — the downward-facing dog. The Dog strengthens, stretches, and tones all parts of your body, but especially your *rhomboids* (the muscles behind your thighs) and *hamstrings* (the muscles on the back of your legs above the knees). The exercise also improves circulation to your head and chest, which helps you feel strong and mentally awake.

Grab your ankle weights and follow these steps:

1. **Get on all fours with your knees directly under your hips and your hands directly below your shoulders.**

   Make sure your fingers are spread wide for support.

2. **Pressing through your palms and the balls of your feet, lift your hips, push your thighs backward, press your sitting bones up to the sky, and move your belly in and up until you're in an upside-down V position (see Figure 7-11a).**

   This is the starting position. Your ears should now be between your arms.

   Stand on the balls of your feet if you can't stretch your hamstrings far enough to keep your feet flat. If your hamstrings and Achilles tendons are tight, feel free to spread your legs a little farther apart.

3. **Inhaling to a count of four, lift your right leg directly behind you toward the ceiling without rotating your hips (see Figure 7-11b).**

   Try to keep your leg straight, and square your hips. Press your hands into the floor and keep your elbows straight. If you're collapsing in your arms, lift up your armpits as if you're shrugging your shoulders.

4. **Exhaling to a count of four, slowly lower your leg to the starting position (see Figure 7-11a).**

If you feel like your arms are working too hard, bend your knees more, pull your belly in, press into your hands, and move your thighs back.

Breathe fully — four counts inhaling and four counts exhaling — as you do this exercise. Alternating legs, perform six to eight repetitions with each leg, pause to rest, and then do six to eight more reps with both legs.

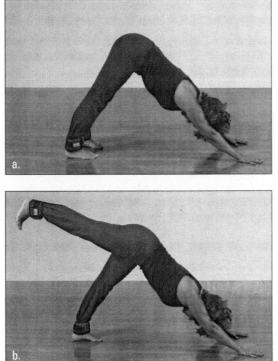

Figure 7-11: Doggedly practice this exercise — it's good for your health.

The Bridge

Maybe you know the old yoga saying: You're as young as your spine is limber. The Bridge is designed to stretch your spine to make it more elastic. The exercise also stretches your rib cage and chest and strengthens your upper back, torso, hamstrings, and calves. As for any wrinkles you may have? Sorry, the bridge can't iron them out.

If you have a lower back problem, do this exercise tentatively at first, and engage your buttocks muscles as you engage your abdominals; this helps stabilize your lower back.

You need your hand weights to cross this bridge; ankle weights are optional. After you've prepared, follow these steps:

1. **Lie on your back with your knees bent, your feet planted flat on the floor, and your palms facing downward while holding the weights on the floor (see Figure 7-12a).**

    This is the starting position. Make sure your lower back is flat against the floor. Look straight up at the ceiling.

2. **Inhaling to a count of four, raise your hips and buttocks to knee height and lift both arms above your head (see Figure 7-12b).**

   Your hands should move 180 degrees to the floor behind you. Press down into your feet as you lift your hips and buttocks, and rely on your shoulders to bear most of the burden.

   If you feel any discomfort in your shoulders, neck, or arms, lift your arms halfway.

3. **Exhaling to a count of four, lower your back to the floor one vertebra at a time and bring your arms forward and back down to the starting position (see Figure 7-12a).**

Keep your tailbone down and your abdominal core strong to take the strain off your lower back during this exercise. And keep your knees stable and in their starting position; they shouldn't wobble.

Do this exercise six to eight times, pause to rest, and then do it six to eight more times.

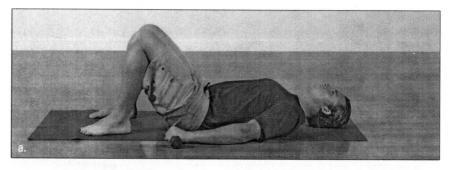

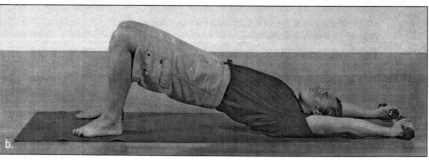

Figure 7-12:
The Bridge aims to make your spine more elastic.

The Frog

It takes some pretty limber muscles to jump from lily pad to lily pad, which is why frogs are good models for yoga-with-weights exercises. This particular exercise, aptly named the Frog, opens up, stretches, and relaxes your groin, hips, and pelvis. It also lengthens your spine. You'll feel your blood coursing through your body as you do the Frog.

Strap on your ankle weights for this exercise and follow these steps:

1. **Lie on your back and, with your knees bent and spread wide, lift your legs to your chest so you can hold your feet, ankles, or calves (see Figure 7-13a).**

   This is the starting position. Draw your belly in and up for support. The bottom of your spine should feel elongated.

   If your knees or inner groin muscles feel tight, extend your legs halfway. You can also hold your inner thighs rather than your feet, ankles, or calves.

2. **Exhaling slowly to a count of four, straighten your right leg as far as you comfortably can while still holding your toes, calves, or ankles (see Figure 7-13b).**

   Pull your belly in; this exercise works your belly muscles, which you need to support your legs and keep them from getting overextended.

   Don't lift your back off the floor or rock your body from side to side.

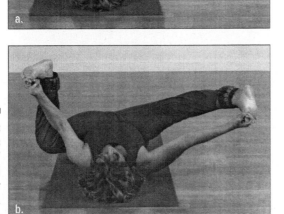

Figure 7-13: The Frog is a hoppin' good exercise for your torso.

3. **Inhaling slowly to a count of four, return your right leg to the starting position (see Figure 7-13a).**

Do this exercise six to eight times with each leg, pause to rest, and then do another six to eight repetitions with each leg.

The Zen

Your Balanced Workout is over — time to relax and enjoy how great your workout has made you feel. As you do this last cool-down exercise, feel the gentle rise and fall of your breath. In yoga, transitions are always important. During this exercise, see if you can make a smooth transition from exercising to whatever activity you want to do next.

You need ankle weights for this exercise, but don't put them on. Follow these steps:

1. **Lie on your back with your ankle weights resting on your diaphragm (see Figure 7-14).**

   The weight is to make you aware of your breathing.

2. **Take in eight to ten Balancing Breaths.**

   Taking Balancing Breaths is a great way to relax (for more detail, see Chapter 4).

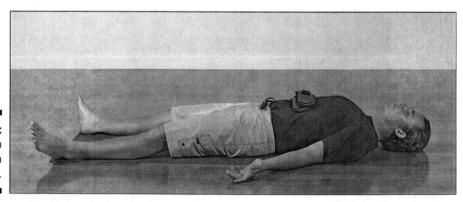

Figure 7-14: Time to relax with the Zen.

Ending Meditation

We recommend that you engage in a moment or two of silent meditation at the end of your workout. A meditation session at the end of a workout brings everything together. It quiets your body and brings closure so you can start afresh with whatever you want to do next in your day (or your night if you're a night-owl yoga-with-weights practitioner). Chapter 6 explains meditation techniques. We encourage you to read that chapter and find a meditation technique that you enjoy and benefit from.

Part II
Mastering the Basics

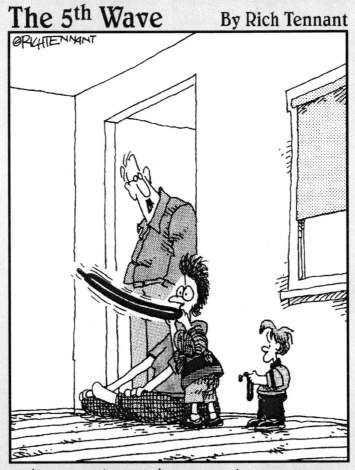

The 5th Wave   By Rich Tennant

"C'mon kids! We've asked you not to do that when your mom's doing her deep breathing exercises."

In this part . . .

*T*ake a deep breath before you start reading Part II, because after you read this part, your breathing will never be the same. You'll understand what a deep breath really feels like.

Part II looks into yoga-with-weights breathing techniques and explores the mental side of yoga with weights — how to break the mental barriers that keep you from exercising and how to quiet and calm your mind. You also practice some warm-up techniques that prepare you to dive into exercises that lead you to a healthy lifestyle. When you're warmed up and ready, tackle the Balanced Workout (see Chapter 7), which we designed to tone your entire body in one workout session.

Chapter 8

Waking Up Your Mind and Body: The Energy Workout

*W*hen you start to feel listless in the afternoon or early evening, forgo the cup of coffee or the sugar-filled snack and do the body shaping, mentally awakening exercises in this chapter instead. Your body will respond in positive ways after you do this energy-boosting workout a few times. You'll feel fitter and more energized as the exercises recharge your spiritual batteries.

The yoga-with-weights exercises in this chapter really get your body moving. We designed these exercises to benefit your circulation and nervous system, allow you to let go of your anxieties, and help you de-stress. The deep breathing brings calm and quiet to help you deal with stress, which gives you more energy and sharpens your senses. You'll discover a keener awareness of the world around you. You'll feel refreshed and renewed.

It takes 20 to 30 minutes to do the Energy Workout. If you perform these exercises several times each week, you'll start to notice your overall energy level improving; your memory sharpening because you aren't tired or stressed out; and your sleep deepening so you feel more relaxed, sharp, and clear throughout the day. You'll create the mental alertness and energy necessary to complete the daily activities that you want to do, and you won't get frustrated or tired as often. These exercises can be a mini-break that makes a positive difference in how you feel — and they take only a few minutes of your day.

Practice the exercises in the Energy Workout with thoughtfulness and care. Don't push yourself too far; take the time to feel your muscles at work, and understand where your exercise limits are. Breathing is an essential element in all the workouts we provide, but especially in this one because of the demand you place on your body. In this workout, you use the Ocean Breath, which you can read about in Chapter 4. This kind of breathing maximizes the potential of your upper chest for breathing and exercising.

The Chair

The Chair is a total-body strengthening exercise that particularly benefits your shoulders, arms, and legs and also exercises your buttocks, abs, and hamstrings. As you do it, press into the ground on all four corners of your feet as you raise and lower the weights.

You need hand weights for this exercise. When you're ready, follow these steps:

1. **Stand with your feet below your hips, your toes pointing forward, and the weights held at your sides with your palms facing inward (see Figure 8-1a).**

   This is the starting position. Draw your belly in and up and your tailbone down for support.

2. **As you inhale to a count of four, sit on an imaginary seat, and slowly raise your arms above your shoulders until they align with your ears (see Figure 8-1b).**

   Raise your arms in front of your body, keeping your palms inward. Imagine that a chair is behind you and you're touching it with your buttocks.

   If your knees bother you, don't crouch as far; take your tailbone down and pull your belly in more. You can also raise your arms only to shoulder height if you have trouble lifting the weights.

3. **As you exhale to a count of four, stand up and slowly lower the weights back to the starting position (see Figure 8-1a).**

Be patient as you do this exercise — let the rhythm of your breathing lift you up and lower you down. As long as you focus on your breathing, you won't throw the weights upward. Inflate your body as you breathe in, letting the intake of air raise your arms as if someone were blowing you up like a balloon.

Repeat this exercise six to eight times, pause to rest, and then do another six to eight repetitions.

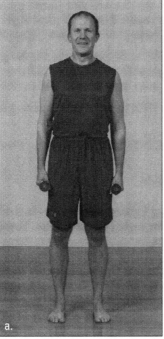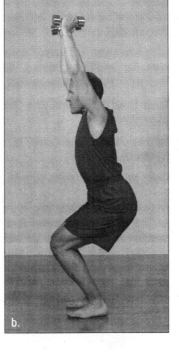

Figure 8-1:
Use the Chair to work your entire body from the (imaginary) seat of your pants.

a.

b.

The Skater

The Skater is an aerobic exercise that works the muscles of your buttocks. By the time you do this exercise twice, you'll be huffing and puffing. The balancing aspect of this exercise fires and stimulates your brain's nerve connections. The Skater is similar to the Chair (see the previous exercise in this workout), but here you lift a leg behind you.

Focus on inhaling and exhaling so you don't do this exercise too fast and throw the weights. Keep your chest open as you inhale and exhale throughout this exercise.

Make sure your ankle weights are strapped on, and grab your hand weights. When you're ready, follow these steps:

1. **Stand with your feet below your hips, your toes pointing forward, and the hand weights at your sides with your palms facing backward (see Figure 8-2a).**

   This is the starting position. Spread your toes wide, pressing hard into the ground through all four corners of both feet — your heels and your toes. You should actively engage both feet. Also, for support, draw your belly in and up and point your tailbone down.

2. **As you inhale to a count of four, lift the weights above your head while you bend your left leg for support and lift your right leg behind you as high as you can without losing balance (see Figure 8-2b).**

   Lift your arms in front of your body until they reach the height of your ears. As you lift, sit back a little bit with your buttocks behind your heel. Feel your buttocks squeezing as your hips are parallel to the floor.

   Keep your leg behind you (don't lift it to your side as a dog does beside a fire hydrant).

3. **As you exhale to a count of four, return to the starting position (see Figure 8-2a).**

   Keep your chest open as you exhale.

If you have trouble balancing, try using lighter weights, or do the exercise without the hand weights and rest your hands on your hips. You can also do this exercise without the ankle weights.

Alternating legs with each repetition, repeat this exercise six to eight times with each leg, pause to rest, and then do another six to eight repetitions with each leg. You're imitating the gliding motion of an ice skater.

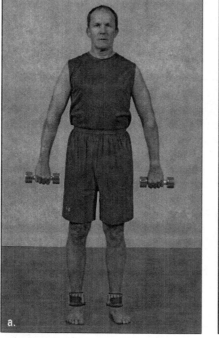
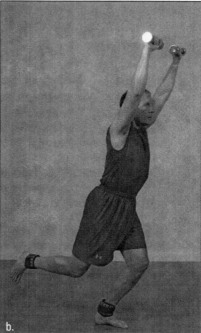

Figure 8-2: Make like the ice skater Michelle Kwan to work your lungs and your buttocks.

The Crow

The Crow is a weighted version of a classic yoga posture that works your buttocks, your upper shoulders, your belly, and your legs. It stretches and conditions your hamstrings and calves and also works your spine. The exercise may seem difficult to do at first, but you can master it with a little practice.

With your ankle weights strapped in place, follow these steps:

1. **Stand with your feet touching or as close to touching as possible, and let your arms fall to your sides.**

2. **Crouch down with your knees parted, put your elbows inside your knees, and rest your hands at shoulder width on the floor (see Figure 8-3a).**

   This is the starting position. You should be squatting deep into your heels. Do your best to keep your heels down while you're in the squatting position.

   If your knees bother you or you have trouble squatting, try squatting halfway. You can also try this exercise without ankle weights if they cause too much trouble for you. Always work at your own level of ability.

3. **As you inhale to a count of four, straighten your left leg and raise your right leg behind you (see Figure 8-3b).**

   Push through your right foot like a swimmer pushing off the side of the pool. Don't rotate your hips; keep them square. Be careful not to kick out your back leg.

   Support yourself with your hands and shoulders as well as your left leg, and sculpt your belly in and up for stability. Keep your supporting leg and your hands flat on the floor.

   If you can't keep your supporting leg straight and maintain your flat hand position, bend your knee a little.

4. **As you exhale to a count of four, lower your extended leg and return to the starting position (see Figure 8-3a).**

Alternating legs, do this exercise six to eight times with each leg, pause to rest, and then do another six to eight reps with each leg.

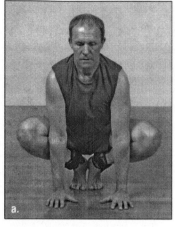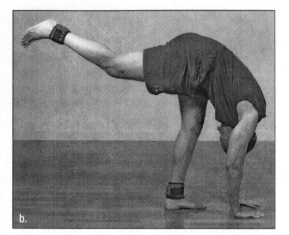

Figure 8-3: The Crow is a full-body exercise that improves your balance and coordination.

The Runner

We call this exercise the Runner because the starting position makes you look like a sprinter in the starting blocks and because you get the feeling of freedom and exhilaration that comes from running in an open field. The exercise strengthens your arm and belly muscles and develops your timing, rhythm, and coordination. The Runner also stretches out your hamstrings, works your legs, and won't upset your allergies like the field.

Strap on your ankle weights and follow these steps:

1. **Start on all fours with your shoulders directly over your wrists and your hips directly over your knees.**

   Spread your fingers wide for support.

   Make sure the inside creases of your elbows face each other. In other words, don't turn your elbows out. If you're limber, you run the risk of tearing a ligament if you turn your elbows out.

2. **Lean back, bringing your heels toward the ground as you draw your knees toward your belly and your buttocks toward your heels (see Figure 8-4a).**

   This is the starting position. Your knees should be deeply bent. Draw your belly in and up and your tailbone down for support.

3. **Exhaling to a count of four, straighten your left leg as you lift your right leg toward the ceiling (see Figure 8-4b).**

   As best you can, keep both legs straight. Focus your eyes on your left knee and shin. Feel your spine stretching.

Remove the ankle weights or wear lighter weights if lifting your leg up high proves too difficult.

4. **Inhaling to a count of four, lower your right leg and return to the starting position (see Figure 8-4a).**

   Look forward as you squat.

Alternating legs, do this exercise six to eight times with each leg, pause to rest, and then do another six to eight reps with each leg.

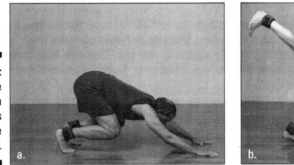
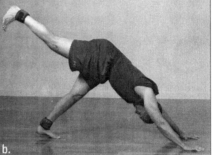

Figure 8-4: Feel the exhilaration of a race as you do the Runner.

The Eye of the Needle

The Eye of the Needle is a squeeze-and-soak exercise, which means it massages your organs (see Chapter 1 for more). The exercise also loosens your spine, opens up your chest and shoulders, and strengthens and conditions your whole upper torso and shoulder-rotation mechanism.

Don't hold your breath in this exercise (be conscious of breathing in and out). Keep your hips over your knees at all times, and remember that your supporting arm should be active the entire time as you look through the Eye of the Needle; don't let this arm go limp.

Grab one hand weight, and make sure your ankle weights are strapped on. When you're ready, follow these steps:

1. **Start on all fours with your hips directly over your knees and your hands on the floor directly below your shoulders; hold a weight in your right hand (see Figure 8-5a).**

   In this position, you should draw your belly below your navel in and up for abdominal stability. Your toes should be pointing straight back.

2. **Inhaling to a count of four, press your left palm down as you slowly raise your right arm up (along with the weight), keeping it straight, and roll your right shoulder back (see Figure 8-5b).**

This is the starting position. Rotate your shoulder and open your chest to the right side as you look toward the ceiling.

3. **Exhaling to a count of four, slowly bring your right hand under and past your body as you stretch out your back and roll onto the backside of your right shoulder (see Figure 8-5c).**

   Your head and the weight should move onto the floor. Feel your back and shoulder stretching as you move the weight onto the floor.

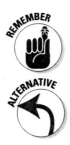

   Watch the weight with your eyes as you roll down. This way, your head flows with the movement of your shoulder and arm. Tuck your chin in slightly to loosen your neck.

   If your shoulders are too tight to roll all the way down, you may want to rest your head on a rolled-up blanket or towel so your neck isn't straining and then gently rotate as far as you can. You can also move your supporting hand forward and out from your body to make the needle loop bigger.

4. **Inhaling to a count of four, return to the starting position (see Figure 8-5b).**

   Pull the weight back through the loop in rhythm with your breathing.

Do this exercise six to eight times with each arm, pause to rest, and then do the exercise six to eight more times with each arm.

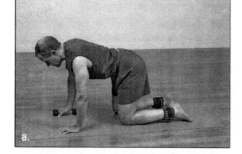
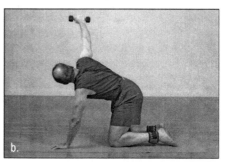
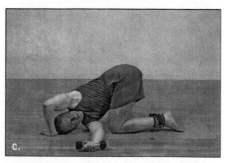

Figure 8-5: You massage your internal organs as you thread the Eye of the Needle.

The Dog to Plank

The Dog to Plank is a powerful upper-body strengthener. This exercise gives you overall strength benefits, which is why you find it in more than one workout (see Chapter 10). It sculpts and tones the entire trunk of your body and also works your buttocks. Along with the strength benefits, the Dog to Plank gives you an endurance exercise with aerobic benefits, and it develops your ability to concentrate. Think the title of the exercise is funny? Well, as you do this exercise, think of how a dog stretches after waking up from a nap, and imagine what your dog is thinking as he watches you.

Make sure you have your ankle weights on, and follow these steps:

1. **Begin on all fours with your hands directly below your shoulders, your knees directly underneath your hips, and your toes planted on the ground (see Figure 8-6a).**

   Spread your fingers wide for support.

2. **Move into the downward-facing dog position by lifting your hips and buttocks as you straighten your legs, bring your thighs back, and move your heels toward the floor.**

   Your ears should be between your arms. Draw your belly in and up and your tailbone down for support.

3. **As you inhale to a count of four, lift your right leg up as high as you can without twisting your hip open (see Figure 8-6b).**

   This is the starting position. Push your leg straight back, and flex your foot to keep it fully engaged — it shouldn't be limp.

4. **As you exhale to a count of four, bring the trunk of your body forward so that your shoulders are over your wrists (see Figure 8-6c).**

   You're in the plank position. Keep your lifted leg parallel to the floor if you're strong enough; otherwise, tap your toe on the floor. You should feel your abdominal and arm muscles working.

   Don't bend your elbows; support your weight through your shoulders and across your back without using your chest muscles.

5. **As you inhale to a count of four, return to the starting position (see Figure 8-6b).**

   Don't lunge backward. Be patient, and move in rhythm with your breathing.

You can do this exercise without ankle weights if you have too much trouble.

Do this exercise six to eight times with each leg, pause to rest, and then do another six to eight repetitions with each leg.

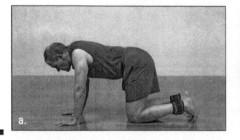

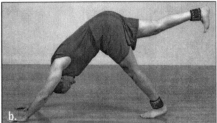

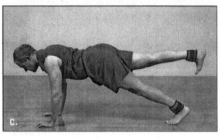

Figure 8-6: The Dog to Plank is a powerful exercise for your upper and lower body.

The Twisted Triangle

The Twisted Triangle is a squeeze-and-soak exercise, which means that it massages your internal organs. Along with warming your insides, it lengthens, tones, stretches, and conditions your legs, back, and spine. Talk about an all-around body conditioner.

If you discover that you're not ready for this exercise, don't rush. Take it slowly. You can injure your lower back if you do the twisting motion in this exercise incorrectly.

You use one hand weight in this exercise. When you're ready, follow these steps:

1. **Stand with your feet as far apart as you comfortably can, with your arms extended straight away from your body forming a straight line with your shoulders (see Figure 8-7a).**

   Make sure you have the weight resting in front of your right foot.

2. **Turn the trunk of your body to face your right leg and, as you bend your right knee, gently lean forward.**

3. **Rest your left hand on the outside of your right foot, and grasp the weight with your right hand (see Figure 8-7b).**

This is the starting position. Draw your belly in and up and your tailbone down for stability and balance.

If you can, square your hips, with your right hip back and your left hip forward. Not everyone can square their hips in this position, however, and if you can't, do your best and don't worry about it.

4. **Exhaling to a count of four, bend your right elbow and lift the weight as you rotate your shoulder and trunk (see Figure 8-7c).**

   Imagine you're an archer pulling back the string of a bow. Twist your trunk, starting at the bottom of your spine and working your way up, one vertebra at a time. Lift your head to the right with the weight as you twist.

   Your left hand should remain by your right foot as you lift. Press down into the balls of your feet for balance and stability.

5. **Inhaling to a count of four, unwind and lower the weight to the starting position (see Figure 8-7b).**

   Be patient as you return to the starting position. Focusing on your breathing helps you return to the starting position in rhythm. Your left hand should remain by your right foot as you lower.

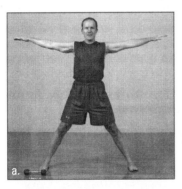
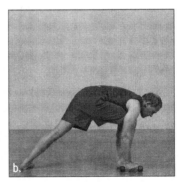

Figure 8-7:
The Twisted
Triangle
conditions
your entire
body.

Try straightening your front leg to stretch your hamstring. If you can't rotate your trunk, lift the weight to exercise your triceps without rotating your shoulder and chest.

Do this exercise six to eight times on each leg, pause to rest, and then do the exercise six to eight more times on each leg.

The Warrior 1

The Warrior I, a relatively simple exercise, is a weighted variation of the classic warrior yoga pose. As you do this exercise, you tap the energy of your heart and feel the strength, honor, and courage of a warrior. On a more practical note, the Warrior I works your biceps and legs.

If you can, keep your hips squared throughout this exercise; neither hipbone should be forward of the other. If squaring your hips is too hard, however, forget it and do your best.

Grab your hand weights and follow these steps:

1. **Standing with your feet below your hips, your toes pointing forward, and the hand weights hanging at your sides with your palms facing inward, step back with your right foot and bend your left leg for support (see Figure 8-8a).**

   This is the lunge position — and the starting position. Turn out your back foot slightly and keep looking forward.

   Your bent knee shouldn't be forward of your ankle. Also, press in with all four corners of your foot.

2. **As you exhale to a count of four, bend your elbows and work your biceps as you lift the weights to shoulder level (see Figure 8-8b).**

   Draw your belly in and up and your tailbone down for support. Keep your elbows locked in; rocking isn't allowed.

3. **As you inhale to a count of four, lower the weights to the starting position (see Figure 8-8a).**

   Don't let your back sag — keep it straight.

Do this exercise six to eight times, pause to rest, and then do six to eight more repetitions.

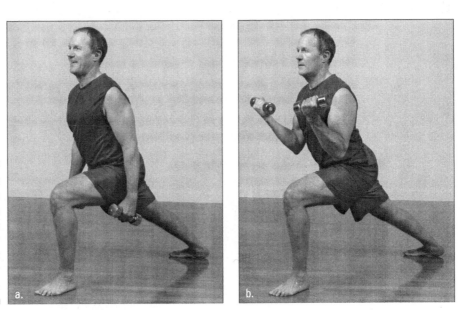

Figure 8-8:
Feel the courage and strength of a warrior while you work your biceps.

The Rise and Shine

The Rise and Shine is a transitional exercise that helps you relax after your strenuous workout. The exercise massages your internal organs and helps you unwind. Imagine you're greeting the morning sun as you do this exercise, feeling its warm rays relaxing your body.

Do a yogic Balancing Breath as you do this exercise (Chapter 4 explains the yoga breaths). Don't rush; take your time and relax.

You need both hand weights for this exercise. When you're ready, follow these steps:

1. **Crouch with your feet about 6 inches apart, your buttocks behind your heels, your elbows outside of your knees, and the weights in your hands with your palms turned inward (see Figure 8-9a).**

   This is the starting position. You should be looking slightly downward. Keep your toes pointing straight ahead throughout this exercise.

2. **As you inhale, pull your belly in and press down through your feet as you rise to a standing position and extend your arms away from your body to the T position (see Figure 8-9b).**

   Your palms should be facing downward at this point.

3. **Continue to inhale as you turn your palms upward and bring your arms together above your head, looking up as you do so (Figure 8-9c).**

Steps 2 and 3 should be one continuous motion.

4. **As you exhale, slowly lower your arms, turn your palms downward again, and return to the starting position (see Figure 8-9a).**

Feel your body deflating as you exhale; slowly lower yourself to the ground in rhythm with your breathing.

Repeat this exercise six to eight times.

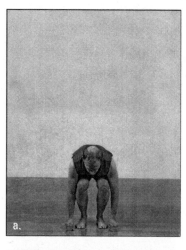
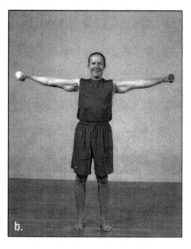
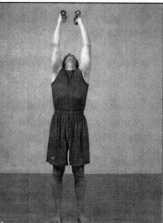

Figure 8-9: Greet the morning sun and say goodbye to your high-energy workout as you do the Rise and Shine.

Ending Meditation

Consider sitting quietly for a moment of meditation after you finish the Energy Workout (Chapter 6 explains meditation techniques in detail). Silent meditation is an excellent way to bring finality to your workout. It calms your body and mind and prepares you for your next activity, whatever it may be.

Chapter 9

Taking It Easy: The Restorative Workout

In This Chapter

▶ Increasing your energy level

▶ Boosting your metabolic rate

▶ Alleviating the stress you carry

▶ Improving your circulation

*I*f you're like most people, you have 101 things to do during your busy day. The Restorative Workout is designed to not only give you the energy to complete your tasks, but also to do them energetically and enthusiastically. The Restorative Workout is the perfect antidote to stress — it leaves you feeling free and unencumbered afterward.

Great, you have the energy for your day . . . but what about the time you don't seem to have? In the 30 minutes it takes you to order a pizza and have it delivered or to make cookies for snacks, you can complete this workout for a boost of energy. You get the energy you need to keep going — and you take a giant step toward getting in shape. You recover the energy you need for your day without having to rely on high-octane sugar snacks or starchy foods. The exercises in this workout give you a kick-start and help you to meet your fitness goals.

If you practice the exercises in the Restorative Workout every other day, you'll stimulate your circulation and your metabolic rate. These exercises keep you moving while giving you the calm, steady energy and equanimity that makes you feel great.

TIP

Try doing these exercises before a party or other special event when you want to feel and look your best and have an alert, stress-free, and bright state of mind.

REMEMBER

For the Restorative Workout, you should use the Complete Breath, which is a deep, relaxing breath. You can discover more about it in Chapter 4.

The Child's Pose

The Child's Pose is a weighted variation of a classic yoga pose. The exercise relaxes your back, head, neck, and shoulders and stretches your spine and *quads* — the muscles of your upper legs. Your body should feel warmed up after working these areas. Besides working your muscles, this introspective exercise can help you collect your thoughts and achieve a state of repose. It massages your intestines to help with digestion and elimination, and you can feel energy passing along your spine to your forehead.

You need hand weights for this exercise. When you're ready, follow these steps:

1. **Starting on your knees and holding the weights at your sides — palms facing backward — touch your feet together, widen your knees, and rest your buttocks on your heels.**

2. **Slowly lean forward, resting your mid-section on your thighs and touching your forehead to the floor (see Figure 9-1a).**

   This is the starting position. Your arms should be extended past your feet with your palms facing upward. Feel your spine stretching and your mid-section resting on your thighs. Don't shrug your shoulders — spread them wide.

   If you have trouble touching your forehead to the floor, spread your knees wider and lower your forehead as far as you can. If you feel uncomfortable resting your buttocks on your heels, try putting a pillow or rolled-up mat under your buttocks. Put a folded blanket under your knees if you feel uncomfortable there. You can also do this exercise without the weights.

3. **Inhale to a count of four as you raise your arms behind you to back-level (see Figure 9-1b).**

   Lift your arms slowly toward the ceiling — don't jerk them, or you may hurt your neck. Draw your belly in and up and your tailbone down for stability.

4. **Exhale to a count of four as you slowly lower the weights to the floor and return to the starting position (see Figure 9-1a).**

Raise and lower your arms in rhythm with your breathing — four counts in and four counts out. Try to keep your buttocks on or close to your heels throughout this exercise.

Do this exercise six to eight times, pause to rest, and then do another six to eight repetitions.

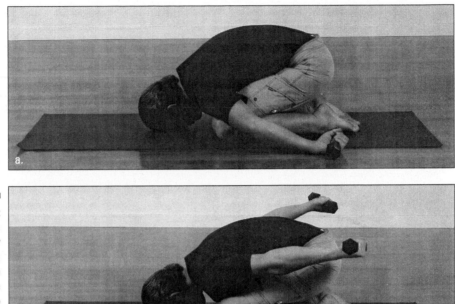

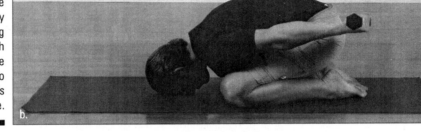

Figure 9-1:
Feel the
energy
surging
through
your spine
as you do
the Child's
Pose.

The Lion

You may not realize it, but you hold tension in your face and jaw. The Lion, a classic yoga exercise to which we've added weights, is designed to release this tension — and to amuse anyone who's in the room while you do it. *Warning:* You make a funny face in this exercise. The Lion also opens up your shoulders, widens your collarbone, and strengthens your spine.

You need your hand weights and ankle weights to become king or queen of the gym. Follow these steps:

1. **Sit comfortably in a cross-legged position with the ankle weights resting on your thighs; rest the hand weights on the ground alongside your body, with your palms facing backward (see Figure 9-2a).**

   This is the starting position. Your spine should be erect, and your ankles should be aligned with your heels. The ankle weights help anchor you during the exercise.

   If you can't sit this way comfortably, sit on a pillow or mat.

2. **Exhaling to a count of four, lift the hand weights forward to ear height, making 90-degree angles with your bent arms.**

3. **With the last of your breath, thrust out your tongue and say "ah"(see Figure 9-2b).**

   Lower your jaw and stick your tongue out — don't be shy. Make the "ah" sound, a slight growling noise. This is the only exercise in this book for which you emit a sound.

4. **Inhaling to a count of four, lower the hand weights down to your sides and close your mouth (pull your tongue in first) to return to the starting position (see Figure 9-2a).**

   Take a moment to enjoy how tension-free your face and jaw feel.

Do this exercise six to eight times, take a rest, and then do it another six to eight times.

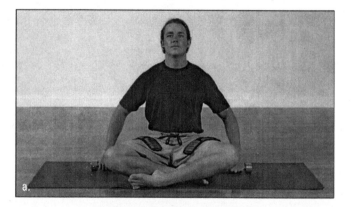

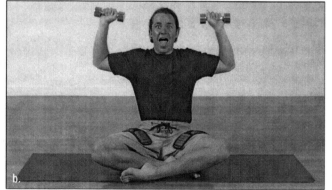

Figure 9-2:
Make like a
kid on the
playground
to release
tension in
your face.

The Pigeon

Many people, especially men, are tight in the hip and groin areas, and the Pigeon is designed to loosen these areas. The Pigeon stretches and expands your hips and inner-thigh muscles by opening up your entire pelvic girdle. It also stretches and lengthens your spine and exercises your biceps.

You need one hand weight for this exercise. Grab it and follow these steps:

1. **From the kneeling position, slide your left leg back and tuck your right heel under your left frontal hip bone (see Figure 9-3a).**

   Keep your hips squared, and try not to drag your left hip backward in this pose. You can bend your left leg slightly; it doesn't have to be straight. Make sure you point your toes.

2. **Slowly lower your elbows to the floor, and rest your trunk on your right thigh.**

   Don't bounce as you drop down — slowly and carefully lower yourself to the floor. Lower yourself as far as you comfortably can if you can't go all the way.

   If your groin or your quad muscle is too tight to do this exercise, place a blanket or folded-up mat under your right buttock or thigh. If you can't lean all the way to the floor, lean halfway and support yourself with one arm.

   Draw your belly in and up and your tailbone down for support. If you feel a pain in your knee, it could be because you're not supporting yourself correctly with the muscles of your belly. This exercise is meant to open up your hips and groin, not stretch your knee.

3. **Grasp the weight in your right hand, keeping your palm face upward (see Figure 9-3b).**

   This is the starting position.

4. **Exhaling to a count of four, bend your right elbow into a bicep curl (see Figure 9-3c).**

   Cross your right hand in front of you as you bend your elbow. Focus on your breathing and feel your thigh, hips, and groin stretching.

5. **Inhaling to a count of four, lower the weight to the starting position (see Figure 9-3b).**

   When you lower the weight, it should land close to your left hand, not below your right shoulder.

Alternating arms and legs, do this exercise six to eight times, pause to rest, and then do another six to eight repetitions, alternating arms and legs.

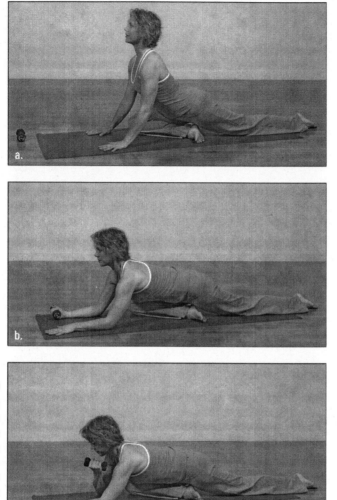

Figure 9-3:
The Pigeon
stretches
your hips
and groin
and gives
your biceps
a workout.

The Sphinx

The Sphinx is a very relaxing exercise that requires concentration. In classic yoga (without weights), the pose is considered the "pose of wisdom," because you look through your third eye — your intuitive and instinctive center. Along with its centering powers, the Sphinx stretches and loosens your head and neck.

The Sphinx is for your neck, not your shoulders. Keep your shoulders square, and don't twist your spine during this exercise.

Strap on your ankle weights and follow these steps:

1. **Lie on your stomach with your elbows under your shoulders — your forearms, wrists, and palms should be flat on the ground — and your chin up (see Figure 9-4a).**

   This is the starting position. Look straight ahead — not up or down. Spread your fingers wide for stability and support.

   If you have difficulty rising onto your elbows without moving your shoulders, simply place your arms farther away from your body and raise your head to a comfortable level.

2. **Inhaling to a count of four, bend your left knee perpendicular to your body as you look over your left shoulder (see Figure 9-4b).**

   Lift your foot over your knee. Turn your head as far as you can without moving your shoulders. Time the movement of your head and leg so that they finish moving at the same time.

3. **Exhaling to a count of four, lower your leg and turn your head back to the starting position (see Figure 9-4a).**

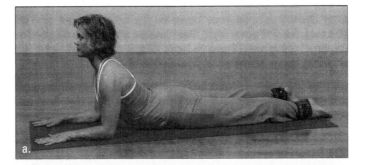

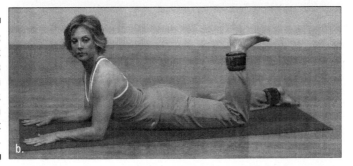

Figure 9-4:
The Sphinx releases tension in your neck as you turn to the left and right.

As you turn your head, look out of the corner of your eyes at your foot, but don't turn your head to look at your foot. When you return to the starting position, look straight ahead. Feel your neck stretching and twisting.

Alternating shoulders, do this exercise six to eight times with each shoulder, pause to rest, and then do another six to eight repetitions with each shoulder.

The Big Ease

Are the exercises in the workout up to this point leaving you sore or tired? Leave it to the Big Ease to iron out your kinks and help you relax. We call it the Big Ease because it's easy to do and it eases your body. The exercise relaxes your hips and stretches all the muscles in the side of your trunk and torso. It also lengthens your quadriceps muscles and releases tension in your hips, neck, and shoulders. You'll enjoy breathing more fully into your chest and lungs as you do this exercise; just don't fall asleep!

You need one hand weight and both ankle weights for this exercise. After you grab the necessary weights, follow these steps:

1. **Sit in a cross-legged position with your feet pulled in and the ankle weights resting on your inner thighs.**

   Resting the weights on your inner thighs helps loosen and warm your thighs and anchor your legs. Your ankles should be aligned with your heels, one heel placed right in front of the other and right in front of your pubic bone. Make sure your spine is erect.

   If you can't sit cross-legged because you feel tight, sit on a pillow or folded-up mat. Doing so relaxes your inner-thigh area and allows your knees to rest more comfortably.

2. **Grab the hand weight with your left hand, and place your right hand on the floor for support (see Figure 9-5a).**

   This is the starting position. Center your shoulders over your hips.

3. **Inhaling to a count of four, lift your left hand over the crown of your head as you feel the side of your body stretching; look toward your right side and gently look down (see Figure 9-5b).**

   Stretch as far as you can with the side of your body without turning your shoulders or leaning forward.

   In this position, you can really feel the advantage of doing yoga with weights, because the weight permits you to stretch farther.

   Don't rush during this exercise. Move the weight slowly without throwing it over your head. You don't want the weight to stretch you too far.

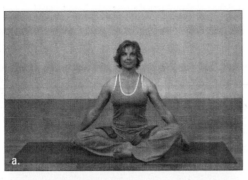

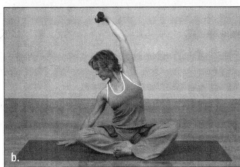

Figure 9-5:
The Big
Ease irons
out the kinks
in your body
and helps
you to relax.

4. **Exhaling to a count of four, return to the starting position (see Figure 9-5a).**

   You can relax your head and look slightly downward to take the tension out of your neck and head, but remember not to lean forward. Draw your belly in and up to help support the weight of your trunk and shoulders.

Do this exercise six to eight times with each side of your body, pause to rest, and then do another six to eight repetitions with each side of your body.

The Gauge

When you do the Gauge, your legs work like the needle of a gauge, moving up and down (but not around in a full circle, unless you're *really* advanced). You'll feel this exercise mostly in your quads. It also lengthens, tones, and conditions the trunk of your body and your arms.

You need both hand weights and ankle weights for this exercise. When you're ready, follow these steps:

1. **Lie on your back with your knees bent and your ankles underneath your knees, and hold the hand weights at your sides with your palms facing downward.**

   Make sure your feet are flat on the ground and as wide apart as your hips.

2. **Straighten your right leg to a 45-degree angle (see Figure 9-6a).**

   This is the starting position.

   Draw your belly in and up and your tailbone down for support. Don't let your abdominal muscles release during the exercise.

3. **Inhaling to a count of four, raise your right leg straight up to a 90-degree angle as you lift the hand weights in a half-circle to the floor behind you (see Figure 9-6b).**

   Don't throw the weights behind you; raise them slowly and consciously. Press into all four corners of your left foot as you lift. Flex your lifted foot so that the bottom is parallel to the ceiling.

   If your shoulders are too stiff, you can lift the hand weights halfway behind your head. If you feel discomfort in your lower back, try this exercise without any hand or ankle weights.

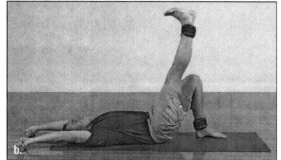

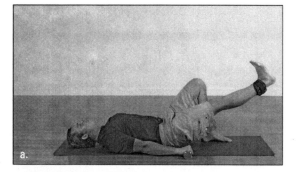

Figure 9-6:
You can feel
the Gauge
deep in
your legs
and core.

4. **Exhaling to a count of four, lower your right leg back to a 45-degree angle and bring your arms back over and down to the starting position (see Figure 9-6a).**

   Time this step so that your leg and your arms arrive at the starting position at the same time. Move the weights as fluidly and rhythmically as possible with the action of your legs.

Do this exercise six to eight times with each leg, pause to rest, and then do another six to eight repetitions with each leg.

The Twister

No, the Twister doesn't mean you need to plan a party and call your friends. This Twister is a squeeze-and-soak exercise, which means that it massages and squeezes your inner organs. The Twister strengthens and tones your waistline, legs, back, and abs. And in order to make you the best twister at your next party, this exercise works your spine to give it more flexibility.

You need both hand weights and ankle weights for this exercise. Follow these steps to get going:

1. **Lie on your back with your knees bent and tucked together high into your chest and your arms straight out from your shoulders in a T position; hold the hand weights with your palms facing upward (see Figure 9-7a).**

   This is the starting position. The higher into your chest you can tuck your knees, the better. Flex and press through all four corners of your feet.

   Holding the hand weights in the T position works as a counterbalance, and the position keeps your collarbones and shoulder blades wide so you have a greater range of motion from side to side.

2. **Exhaling to a count of four, slowly move your joined knees to the right until your right knee touches the floor (see Figure 9-7b).**

   Make sure your knees are stacked one on top of the other. Don't drop your legs; control their downward motion by concentrating on your four-count breathing.

   As you move your legs to one side, keep your opposite shoulder on the ground.

3. **Inhaling to a count of four, slowly lift your joined knees back to the starting position (see Figure 9-7a).**

   Sculpt your belly in and up as you lift. By contracting your abdominal muscles and keeping them engaged, you give support to your legs.

If you experience discomfort in your lower back, do this exercise without the ankle weights.

Do this exercise six to eight times on each side of your body, pause to rest, and then do another six to eight repetitions on each side of your body.

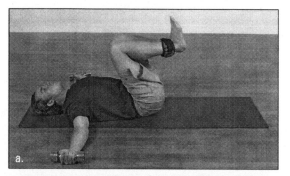

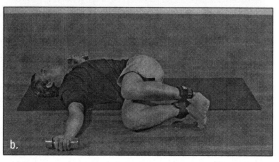

Figure 9-7:
To get the most out of the Twister, move and breathe slowly and consciously.

The Plow

A farming plow has only one or two specific uses . . . you plow the ground and plant your seeds. The yoga-with-weights Plow, however, serves many functions for your body. It loosens your lower back, extends your legs, releases your hamstrings, and exercises your abdominal muscles. You'll feel your spine and lower back stretching in this exercise. The Plow also reverses the blood flow in your legs, which is good for circulation and reducing bloating and water retention in your ankles.

Strap on your ankle weights and grab both hand weights for this exercise and follow these steps:

1. **Lie on your back with your legs raised straight, your feet and knees above your hips, and your hands at your sides holding the hand weights, palms turned downward (see Figure 9-8a).**

This is the starting position.

Make sure your feet are *yoga feet* — they should be flexed and engaged, and you should be pressing into all four corners of each foot. At all times during this exercise, make sure your abdominal muscles, which help support your legs, are engaged.

2. **Exhaling to a count of four and keeping your legs straight, slowly lift your buttocks off the floor, and extend your legs so that your feet are above your head, not your hips (see Figure 9-8b).**

The hand weights act as anchors so you can stretch your back. Feel a gentle squeeze and lift in your buttocks.

If you can't extend your legs above your head, move them as far as you comfortably can. If you can't straighten your legs, do this exercise with your knees bent.

3. **Inhaling to a count of four, return to the starting position (see Figure 9-8a).**

Don't bounce as you do this exercise; move your legs slowly and consciously as you focus on your breathing.

Do this exercise six to eight times, pause to rest, and then do another six to eight repetitions.

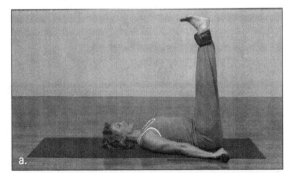

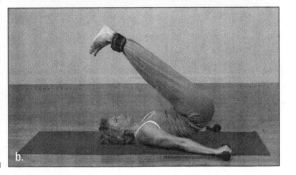

Figure 9-8:
Feel your lower back stretching and your buttocks squeezing when you pull the Plow.

The Serenity

The Serenity is a relaxing pose designed to transition you from the Restorative Workout to the rest of your day. You should understand that gravity is your friend and feel the heaviness of your body resting. The natural force is removing the fatigue from your body. Feel the waters of your mind coming to a standstill — try imagining that you're a sun-warmed rock in the middle of a rushing stream.

You need a single ankle weight for this exercise. When you're ready, follow these steps:

1. **Lie on your back with the ankle weight resting across your abdomen and your arms in a T position, palms facing upward (see Figure 9-9).**

   This is the starting (and ending) position. Make sure your legs are straight.

2. **Using Abdominal Breaths, slowly inhale to four counts.**

   Feel the gentle rounding and fullness of your belly as you breathe in deeply. (For more on Abdominal Breaths, refer to Chapter 4.)

3. **Slowly exhale to six counts.**

   As you exhale, feel your belly deflating toward the floor.

Relax throughout this exercise. Feel your body unwind and loosen up.

The Serenity calls for six to eight abdominal breaths.

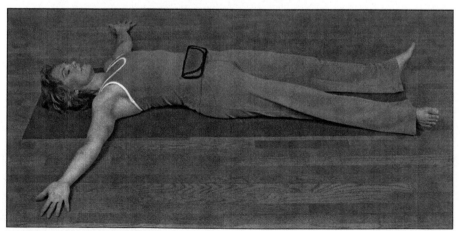

Figure 9-9:
Feel your lower back stretching and your body releasing anxiety and stress.

Ending Meditation

Before you say goodbye to the Restorative Workout and go back to riding rodeo bulls or whatever you plan to do next, engage in a moment or two of silent meditation. Meditation helps you integrate the work you've just done into your body; it gives your body a chance to feel what it has just experienced and absorb the benefits physically and mentally. Chapter 6 explains several meditation techniques. Find a technique you enjoy and do it at the end of this workout.

Chapter 10

Pumping You Up: The Strengthening Workout

- -

In This Chapter

▶ Loosening and then tightening your body and mind

▶ Building strength in your core

▶ Improving your physical stability with balance and coordination

- -

Keeping your body strong and your mind in-tune are the keys to well-being. You have more energy. You're more capable of doing physical activities, and you can maintain your concentration longer. You can resist stress better. You can withstand the daily pressures you have to labor under. When you feel strong, you're more confident. It's much harder to rock the boat emotionally, and the choices you make in your life are more consistent with the quality of life you desire.

The exercises in this workout strengthen your muscles and provide you with a greater sense of physical and mental stability. They give you a greater sense of balance, which leads to an increase in confidence. By practicing these exercises and focusing on your breathing, you can create a renewed sense of confidence and strength within. We call this new strength *stability* — it's a resource that comes alive just when you need it. We encourage you to take the dive with a big smile and find out what's waiting for you on the other side.

The exercises in the Strengthening Workout are a little harder to do because they're designed to build strength. Don't push yourself too hard in the beginning. The first step takes you to the next, which takes you to the next, and so on. All you have to do is stay in the moment with each exercise. You need to work at your own level of ability. Take it slow and steady, maintaining your rhythmic deep breathing throughout this workout. If an exercise doesn't feel right, simply skip over it and go to the next exercise. As you build your strength, you'll eventually be able to do all the exercises in the Strengthening Workout with confidence and ease.

For the Strengthening Workout, you should take deep, slow Complete Breaths. Chapter 4 explains the Complete Breath and other breathing techniques.

The Lightning Bolt

The Lightning Bolt is an energy pose that gives your body the get-up-and-go it needs to continue the Strengthening Workout. It strengthens your legs; it develops range of motion in your shoulders, hips, and pelvic girdle; and it helps you develop balancing skills. Get ready to feel a surge of energy as you do this exercise.

Pick up your hand weights and follow these steps:

1. **Stand with your legs below your hips, holding the weights above your head with your arms straight and the palms of your hands facing one another (see Figure 10-1a).**

   This is the starting position.

2. **Exhaling to a count of four, bend your knees and squat as you lower the weights to the floor in front of you (see Figure 10-1b).**

   As you bring your arms down, keep them straight, and make sure your hands remain facing each other when the weights reach the floor. Your gaze should follow the movement of your body. Look down as you squat, following the weights with your eyes. Draw your belly in and up and your tailbone down as you squat for support.

   Be careful not to lean too far forward with your knees; sit down into the squatting position.

   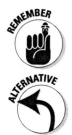

   Squat halfway if you're not ready to go all the way down. If you feel any stiffness in your shoulders, you can take your arms only halfway down as well.

3. **Inhaling to a count of four, push through your feet and rise to the starting position (see Figure 10-1a).**

   Rise slowly and make sure your palms continue to face one another. Concentrate on pushing the ground away from your body, and look up with the weights as you rise.

Be patient. Don't "fall down" as you squat or "jump up" when you rise. Control the rise and fall of the weights, and focus on your breathing.

Do this exercise six to eight times, pause to rest, and then do another six to eight repetitions.

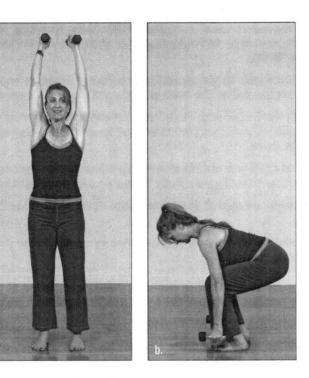

Figure 10-1:
The Lightning Bolt works your legs and loosens your arms and hips.

The Crescent Moon

The Crescent Moon is a lunging exercise that requires balance and concentration. It works your buttocks, thighs, hips, and quads. The exercise can be difficult at first because it requires concentration and muscle strength, but stick with it — you'll improve over time.

Grab your hand weights and follow these steps:

1. **Stand with your feet below your hips, your toes pointing forward, and the weights hanging at your sides with your palms facing inward.**

2. **Step back onto the ball of your right foot, keeping your legs straight and the hand weights at your sides (see Figure 10-2a).**

   This is the starting position. Your shoulders should be squared, and you should gaze straight ahead. Make sure you're resting on the ball of your right foot with your heel raised.

3. **Exhaling to a count of four, gently dip down, bending your left knee to a 90-degree angle and bringing your right knee close to the floor (see Figure 10-2b).**

Draw your belly in and up and your tailbone down for support and stability. Let the pull of the hand weights guide your downward motion.

Stay on the ball of your back foot, and support your weight on all four corners of your front foot. Don't let your front knee roll forward of your ankle when you dip down.

Don't worry if you can dip down only a few inches. Just make sure you concentrate on drawing your belly in and up and your tailbone down.

4. **Inhaling to a count of four, rise to the starting position (see Figure 10-2a).**

Keep your hips as square as possible as you rise to the rhythm of your breathing.

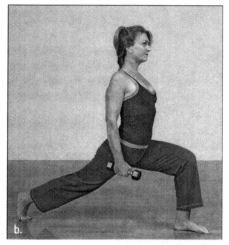

To give yourself an even better workout, bend your elbows at your sides in the starting position and push the hand weights upward from your shoulders as you dip.

Do this exercise six to eight times on each leg, pause to rest, and then do it another six to eight times on each leg.

Figure 10-2:
The Crescent Moon challenges your ability to balance and concentrate.

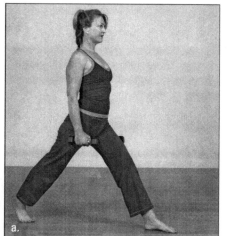

The Dog to Plank

The Dog to Plank appears in more than one workout in this book (see Chapter 8) because it's such a superb, powerful exercise. You could say that it's one of the most strengthening of the strengthening exercises. The exercise sculpts and tones your entire upper body, offers aerobic benefits, and helps you develop the ability to concentrate. Don't give up on this exercise; if you train your mind to do it, your body will follow.

Fasten your ankle weights and follow these steps (if the steps prove too tough at first, you don't have to use the ankle weights):

1. **Begin on all fours with your hands directly below your shoulders, your knees directly underneath your hips, and your toes planted on the ground.**

   Spread your fingers wide for support.

2. **Move into the downward-facing dog position by lifting your hips and buttocks as you straighten your legs, bring your thighs back, and move your heels toward the floor (see Figure 10-3a).**

   Your ears should be between your arms. Draw your belly in and up and your tailbone down for support.

3. **As you inhale to a count of four, lift your right leg up as high as you can without twisting your hip open (see Figure 10-3b).**

   This is the starting position. Push your leg straight back, and flex your foot to keep it fully engaged — it shouldn't be limp.

4. **As you exhale to a count of four, bring the trunk of your body forward so that your shoulders are over your wrists (see Figure 10-3c).**

   You're in the plank position. Keep your lifted leg parallel to the floor if you're strong enough; otherwise, tap your toe on the floor. You should feel your abdominal and arm muscles working.

   Don't bend your elbows; support your weight through your shoulders and across your back without using your chest muscles.

5. **As you inhale to a count of four, return to the starting position (see Figure 10-3b).**

   Don't lunge backward. Be patient, and move in rhythm with your breathing.

Do this exercise six to eight times with each leg, pause to rest, and then do it another six to eight times with each leg.

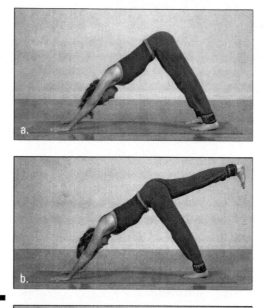

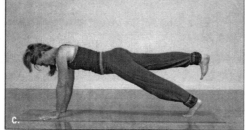

Figure 10-3:
The Dog to Plank is tough, but it gives you a good upper-body workout.

The Side Plank

The Side Plank is an unusual yoga-with-weights exercise in that you work only one side of your body at a time, which presents new challenges for balancing. The exercise opens up your shoulder girdle and strengthens your trunk, shoulders, hips, and pelvis. Much like the Dog to Plank — the previous exercise in this workout — the Side Plank can be a grueling exercise. But like the Dog to Plank, it offers enormous benefits for your mind and body.

You need both ankle weights and one hand weight for this exercise. When you're ready, follow these steps:

1. **Sit on your right hip, and cross your left foot over your right leg, placing your left heel next to your right thigh.**

   Hold the hand weight in your left hand, with your palm facing your body.

2. **Straighten your right arm, pressing onto your right hand as you lift your hip from the floor (see Figure 10-4a).**

   This is the starting position. Press into the foot of your left leg as you lift to help with the burden. The hand weight should be dangling off the ground, and you should be looking at the ground. Your whole body — your shoulder and both legs, as well as your abdominal muscles — supports you here.

3. **As you inhale to a count of four, pull the hand weight above your shoulder as you bend your elbow, drawing your left shoulder blade back and squeezing your shoulder blades together (see Figure 10-4b).**

   Make sure your wrist is above your shoulder. Rotate your gaze with the weight as you open up your trunk.

4. **As you exhale to a count of four, lower the weight to the starting position (see Figure 10-4a).**

   Let the weight guide your arm to the floor; don't throw it down. Follow the weight with your eyes, and stay in tune with your breathing.

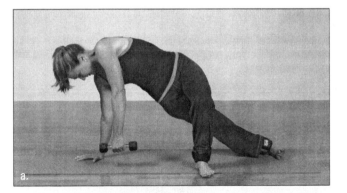

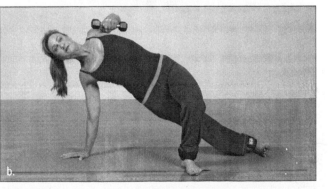

Figure 10-4: The Side Plank makes you solid as a board from head to toe.

If you have trouble with this exercise, do it without the hand weight. You can also support your body with your elbow and forearm rather than your hand.

Do this exercise four to eight times with each arm, pause to rest, and then do another four to eight repetitions with each arm.

The Half Moon

The Half Moon is a pose of concentration and balance that fires the nerves of your brain. The pose is as much about balance and stability as it is about strength. It works every part of your legs and buttocks and also strengthens your arms. The Half Moon will leave your body and mind fully invigorated.

Strap on your ankle weights and follow these steps:

1. **Kneel on your left leg, put your right hand on your right hip, and support your upper body with your left arm; make sure your left wrist is directly under your shoulder.**

   Put padding under your left knee if you need it.

2. **Raise your right leg to the height of your hip, keeping it straight and extended outward, as you open your trunk to the right (see Figure 10-5a).**

   This is the starting position. Sculpt your belly in and up so that your abdominal muscles help support you in this position. You should be looking to your right.

3. **Exhaling to a count of four, lower your right foot to the ground as you turn your head to look down (see Figure 10-5b).**

   Keep your right foot flexed and engaged throughout this step.

   You can lower your right leg halfway if bringing it to the floor is too difficult.

4. **Inhaling to a count of four, raise your right leg and turn your head to the starting position (see Figure 10-5a).**

   Move slowly while you concentrate on the rhythm of your breathing.

Do this exercise six to eight times, pause to rest, and then do another six to eight repetitions.

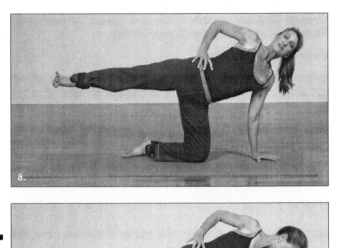

Figure 10-5:
The Half
Moon is a
mental
workout as
well as a
physical
challenge.

The Swimmer

The Swimmer is a right brain–left brain, cross-shifting exercise. Because you work opposite arms and legs, you develop coordination and balance skills. The exercise works your arms, legs, *lats* (the muscles in your upper back), and buttocks. The trunk of your body also gets a workout.

Strap on both ankle weights and grab one hand weight for this exercise. When you're ready, follow these steps:

1. **Get on all fours with your wrists directly below your shoulders and your knees directly under your hips.**

   After you get in this position, grab the hand weight with your left hand and keep it on the ground, directly under your shoulder. Spread the fingers of your right hand for support. Focus your gaze on the fingers of your supporting hand.

   You can roll up a mat or pillow and put it under your supporting hand if you get tired too easily during this exercise. Elevating your hand distributes your weight more evenly across your entire body.

2. **Extend your right leg straight back, and plant the ball and toes of your right foot on the ground (see Figure 10-6a).**

   This is the starting position.

3. **As you inhale to a count of four, raise your left arm and right leg simultaneously to the height of your shoulders and hips (see Figure 10-6b).**

   Keep your eyes on the fingers of your supporting hand so you don't strain your neck.

4. **As you exhale to a count of four, lower your left arm and right leg to the starting position (see Figure 10-6a).**

   Be patient as you lower your arm and leg — don't drop them to the floor.

The more times you do this exercise, the easier it will become to lift the weights.

Alternating arms and legs, do this exercise six to eight times, pause to rest, and then do another six to eight repetitions with each arm and leg.

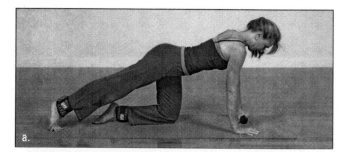

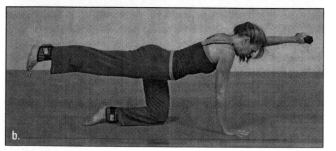

Figure 10-6:
Who said swimming upstream was easy?

The Rabbit

The Rabbit is a restorative pose, so we include it here to help you recharge your batteries. This exercise reinvigorates your back and spine and massages your internal organs.

Grab your ankle weights for this exercise and follow these steps:

1. **Sit with your knees bent so your buttocks are resting on your heels, and place the ankle weights on your thighs (see Figure 10-7a).**

   This is the starting position.

2. **Make the trunk of your body as long as you can make it, and grasp your heels with your hands.**

3. **Lower your trunk onto your thighs (see Figure 10-7b).**

   Tuck your chin gently to keep your airway open. Rest your forehead on the floor if you can. Draw your belly in and up and your tailbone down for support, and let your shoulders widen and stretch.

4. **Feel your back stretching as you take four to eight long, slow breaths.**

   Focus on relaxing while your back stretches.

5. **Raise your trunk to the starting position (see Figure 10-7a).**

Try putting the ankle weights on your back to give yourself a better stretch. You'll need some help from a friend with this variation in order to lay the weights across your back in a way that keeps them in place.

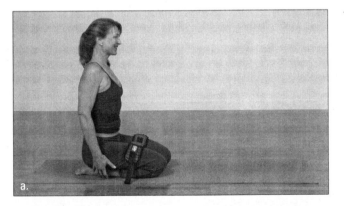

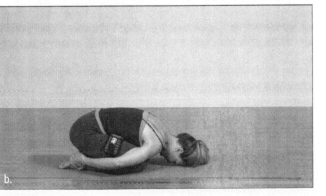

Figure 10-7: Westing in wepose wike a wabbit.

The Dolphin

The Dolphin is a weighted variation of a classic yoga pose. The version we introduce is truly a full-body strengthener. The pose reverses the blood flow in your legs, which is good for circulation and reducing bloating and water retention in your ankles, and exercises your hamstrings, calves, and Achilles tendons. The exercise is also a powerful upper-body builder because you have to support your body with the muscles in your upper half.

Strap on your ankle weights and follow these steps:

1. **Kneel with your elbows below your shoulders, your knees below your hips, your forearms and hands flat on the floor in front of you, and your toes curled onto the floor (see Figure 10-8a).**

   Spread your fingers wide for support.

   Don't let your elbows splay out beyond your shoulders. Doing so can make your shoulders roll in, which can cause injury to your rotator cuff.

2. **Press down into your forearms, hands, and the balls of your feet as you lift your buttocks into the air (see Figure 10-8b).**

   This is the starting position. You should be looking back at your legs. Your head shouldn't touch the floor at any time; let it dangle between your arms and elbows as you press your wrists and forearms downward.

   Press your hands, wrists, and forearms into the floor for support. Support your body with your shoulders as well as your arms and legs. Feel your armpits lifting toward the ceiling and forward toward your hands.

3. **As you inhale to a count of four, extend your right leg directly behind you so it forms a straight line with your torso (see Figure 10-8c).**

   If you feel too much stress on your shoulders, press into your hands, wrists, and forearms to put more weight on those areas.

4. **As you exhale to a count of four, slowly lower your leg to the starting position (see Figure 10-8b).**

Moving your leg slowly is important for your balance. Keep your hips squared; don't turn or wobble them as you lift and lower your leg.

Do this exercise six to eight times on each leg, pause to rest, and then do another six to eight repetitions on each leg.

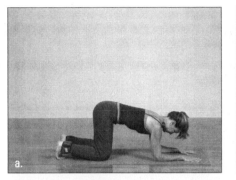
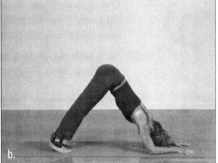

Figure 10-8:
The Dolphin
challenges
your upper
body as
you lift
your legs.

The Lift

Of all the strengthening exercises in this workout, the Lift concentrates the most on strengthening the back of your body — the back of your arms, spine, and legs. The Lift is also a concentration-coordination exercise that challenges your ability to control your body. The Lift squeezes and tones your kidneys and works out the muscles of your abdomen.

You need both hand weights and both ankle weights for this exercise. When you're ready, follow these steps:

1. **Lie flat on your belly with your forehead touching the floor and your arms at your sides holding the hand weights, palms facing upward (see Figure 10-9a).**

   This is the starting position. Shrug your shoulders slightly to move your arm bones into the shoulder girdle. Draw your belly in and up and your tailbone down for support.

2. **As you inhale to a count of four, raise your chin, arms, and legs up into the air as far as you comfortably can (see Figure 10-9b).**

   Feel your entire body working. Your abdominal muscles should bear most of the weight of your body as your trunk supports you.

If you aren't yet strong enough to hold the hand weights in the air, do this exercise without them. Remove the weights from your legs as well if you have too much trouble lifting your legs.

3. **As you exhale to a count of four, lower your lifted parts to the starting position (see Figure 10-9a).**

Concentrate on your breathing every step of the way as you raise and lower your body. Be careful not to raise one leg higher than the other, and remember to engage your abdominal and other core muscles, which prevents your back from being injured in this exercise.

Do this exercise six to eight times, pause to rest, and then do another six to eight repetitions.

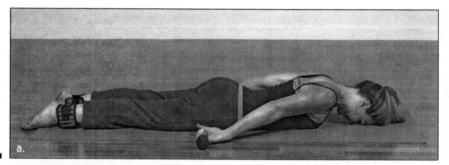

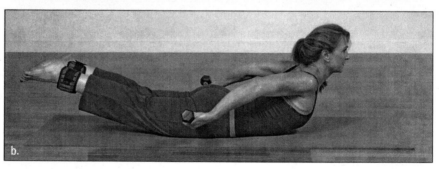

Figure 10-9:
The Lift strengthens the back-side of your body and raises your level of coordination.

Ending Meditation

After you finish the Strengthening Workout, set aside a moment to engage in meditation. A meditation session is like tying a bow on your workout — it signals the end of one activity and the beginning of the next. Meditation teaches you to flow and function with a calm mind. Chapter 6 explains several meditation techniques.

Chapter 11

Releasing Your Athlete Within: The Endurance Workout

In This Chapter

▶ Developing a sustained ability to focus and concentrate

▶ Building your body strength

▶ Fighting through fatigue to cleanse mind and body

---

*W*hen most people think of endurance, they think about being able to go beyond physical limitations or overcoming fatigue. This workout provides exercises and mindfulness practices to help you develop not only your physical strength, but also your mental will to keep going when the going gets tough. Each time you practice these exercises, you develop a little more stamina to endure in a healthy, mindful way.

We believe that the ability to concentrate and focus is an essential part of endurance, so we include exercises in this workout designed to help you concentrate and focus. Sometimes, endurance is simply a matter of putting aside the large and small distractions so you can focus on the task at hand. Other times, endurance is a matter of talking to yourself — of conducting an inner dialogue so you can push ahead through the distractions. When you communicate with yourself, you can remove the obstacles that may be standing in your way. You can walk the forward path in life with an ease that will amaze you.

Using the mind and body techniques in Chapter 5 along with the exercises in this chapter, you can develop the strength and endurance to go the extra mile. You'll discover how to access the power of concentration and inner resilience to meet your mental and physical demands. Endurance training is an opportunity to train your mind while strengthening your body.

 Depending on your level of need and how hard you want to train, we recommend doing the Endurance Workout twice a week. If you're training for a triathlon or other grueling sport, work out three times a week, and alternate on other days with the Strengthening Workout we present in Chapter 10.

Use Ocean Breaths for the Endurance Workout (see Chapter 4) if you want a powerful workout; if you're a beginner, you may want to start with Complete Breaths.

The Tree

The Tree is a variation of a classic yoga pose. Because it requires you to balance, it exercises your ability to concentrate. On the physical side, it stretches the back of your spine and works your triceps. The Tree is a good exercise for women because it works the sometimes-flabby muscles on the back of the arms.

As you do this exercise, it helps to imagine that you're a tree growing sturdy roots in the earth. Focus your energy on your balance, and throughout the exercise, draw your belly in and up and your tailbone down for balance and support.

Grab one hand weight for this exercise and follow these steps:

1. **Stand with your feet below your hips, your toes pointing forward, your hands at your hips, and the weight in your right hand, palm facing inward.**

   Make sure your spine is erect. No slouching allowed!

2. **Using your left hand for assistance, lift your left foot and tuck it into your right inner thigh (see Figure 11-1a).**

   If you can't tuck your foot into your thigh, press it directly above or below your knee, or place it on your right ankle. Imagine that you're attaching your foot to your leg, knee, or ankle by Velcro.

   Press into all four corners of your right foot for stability.

3. **Grab the weight with both hands and move it above and then behind your head while you continue to look forward (see Figure 11-1b).**

   This is the starting position. Bring your armpits back as far as you can; feel them stretching.

4. **Exhaling to a count of four, straighten your arms as you raise the weight over your head (see Figure 11-1c).**

   As best you can, keep your elbows beside your ears as you raise the weight. Press your arms toward the ceiling; don't swing them.

5. **Inhaling to a count of four, bend your elbows back and lower the weight behind your head to the starting position (see Figure 11-1b).**

   Maintain your elbows' positions beside your ears.

If you have trouble balancing, stand next to a wall and press the knee of your bent leg into the wall. This way, you balance without fear of falling and focus on your belly, spine, and arm action.

Repeat this exercise six to eight times on each leg, take a rest, and then do six to eight more repetitions on each leg.

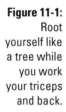

Figure 11-1:
Root
yourself like
a tree while
you work
your triceps
and back.

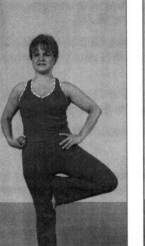 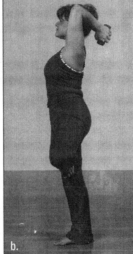 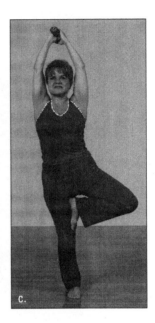

The Dancer

Dancing is a full-body activity that requires physical and mental prowess. The yoga-with-weights Dancer is no different. This exercise helps you develop focus and concentration as it strengthens your biceps, legs, and shoulder girdle. It also allows for a greater range of motion in your shoulders. You'll feel uplifted and stretched like a dancer as you do this exercise.

Take your time with the Dancer. Think of it as a slow dance, not a salsa. If you're patient, you won't lose your balance.

Grab one of your hand weights and follow these steps:

1. **Stand with your feet below your hips, your toes pointing forward, your arms hanging down at your sides, and your right hand holding the weight, palm facing backward.**

2. **Bend your left knee, and reach back for your left foot with your left hand and grasp it (see Figure 11-2a).**

This is the starting position. Bend your right knee ever so slightly, and make sure that all four corners of your right foot are firmly on the floor for stability. To stay balanced, draw your belly in and up for support, and keep your chest and trunk lifted.

If you can't hold your foot, try holding your pants leg. You can also do the exercise with a bent knee or in the standing position.

3. **Inhaling to a count of four, lift the weight in front of your body and then above your shoulder, keeping your arm straight, as you extend your lifted foot behind you (see Figure 11-2b).**

   Move your leg straight behind you; don't lift it to the side like a dog at a fire hydrant. Don't hurl the weight; raise it gently in rhythm with your breathing.

4. **Exhaling to a count of four, lower the weight to your side, and return your lifted foot to the starting position (see Figure 11-2a).**

   Make sure your arm stays straight as you lower the weight in rhythm with your breathing.

Repeat this exercise six to eight times on your right leg, taking a short rest between repetitions, and then do six to eight repetitions on your left leg.

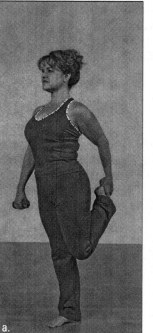
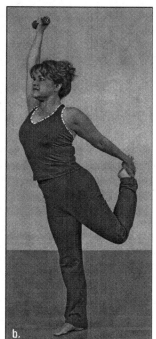

Figure 11-2:
Enjoy a full-body (and mind) workout and the exhilaration of dancing.

a.   b.

The Eagle

The Eagle is an endurance challenge. Although the exercise works your biceps and the muscles of your thighs and legs, it really challenges your mind and ability to balance. The Eagle requires discipline, focus, and concentration.

You need both hand weights for this exercise. When you're ready, follow these steps:

1. **Stand with your feet below your hips, your toes pointing forward, and your arms hanging at your sides, holding the weights with your palms facing forward.**

2. **Sit downward slightly, and lift your left leg and cross it over your right thigh, calf, and ankle (see Figure 11-3a).**

   This is the starting position. You're in the classic yoga eagle pose. Challenging, isn't it? Here are some tips to get into and stay in this pose:

   - Pull your tailbone gently down toward the floor and slightly forward.

   - Bend your right leg at the same time as you sit downward.

   - Put one knee directly in front of the other, draping it over the top of the supporting knee.

   - Point your toes down and back toward the calf of your bent leg.

   - Squeeze your inner thighs together.

   Feel your spine gently stretching and lengthening. Make sure that you're looking straight ahead, your shoulders are squared, and your elbows are slightly bent.

   If you can't get into this difficult pose, don't wrap your leg all the way around. Take your leg halfway around, or simply cross your legs. You can also put your left toe down on the other side of your right foot. This way, you can take the toe off the floor to check your balance without too much effort.

3. **Exhaling to a count of four, bend your elbows and curl your arms to lift the weights (see Figure 11-3b).**

   Feel your upper arms working. Keep your elbows against your body as you raise the weights. Squeeze your thighs for support.

4. **Inhaling to a count of four, lower your arms to the starting position (see Figure 11-3a).**

   Make sure your elbows don't stray from your body on the way down. Feel the burn in your right thigh as you continue to squeeze it for support.

Keep both your feet fully engaged throughout this exercise; be sure to press through all four corners of each foot. Concentrating on your feet helps your balance.

Repeat this exercise six to eight times on each leg, take a rest, and then do six to eight more repetitions on each leg.

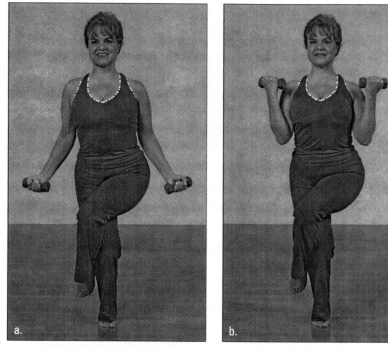

Figure 11-3:
The Eagle is a demanding yoga pose that builds endurance.

a.   b.

The Russian Dancer

The Russian Dancer is an exercise that helps build strength, stamina, and endurance. It tones and conditions your legs and gently engages your pelvic region. The exercise is relatively easy to do, but it gives you a good workout and tests your endurance. You'll feel like you danced up a storm all night long after you finish!

You need both hand and ankle weights for this exercise. When you're ready, follow these steps:

1. **Stand with your feet below your hips, your toes pointing forward, and your arms dangling at your sides, holding the hand weights with your palms facing inward.**

   This is the starting position. Look straight ahead.

2. **Inhaling to a count of four, lift your right knee to the height of your hips (see Figure 11-4a).**

   Your knee should be bent at a 90-degree angle, with your foot below your knee.

3. **Exhaling to a count of four, press your right heel away from your body and straighten your leg (see Figure 11-4b).**

   Your supporting leg should be straight, but if you can't keep it straight, that's okay. Let your knee bend gently in the beginning until you're flexible and strong enough to keep it straight.

   Flex your foot, and really push your leg out.

4. **Inhaling to a count of four, return your right leg to the bent-knee position (see Figure 11-4a).**

5. **Exhaling to a count of four, lower your right leg to the starting position (see Step 1).**

Alternating legs, repeat this exercise six to eight times with each leg, take a rest, and then do six to eight more repetitions with each leg.

Figure 11-4:
The Russian Dancer strengthens your legs and heightens your concentration.

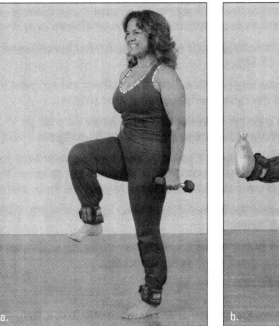
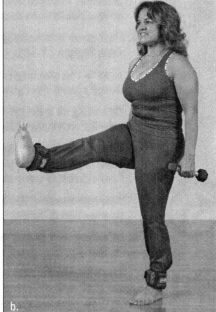

The Road Runner

The Road Runner starts you in the same position as a runner in the starting blocks and works the same muscles as running does. What's more, you get the same feeling of exhilaration that a runner gets when crossing the finish line in first place. This exercise works your hamstrings, legs, and belly muscles and strengthens your entire upper torso. It also helps you develop rhythm and coordination. You can test your endurance and find the strength and focus to run that extra mile in any area of your life.

Be sure to breathe fully and rhythmically throughout this exercise. Feel the air filling your lungs all the way to your collarbones.

Strap on both ankle weights and follow these steps:

1. **Start on all fours with your shoulders directly over your wrists, your hips directly over your knees, and your toes and the balls of your feet touching the ground.**

   Spread your fingers wide for support.

   People who have elastic muscles sometimes turn their elbows out in this posture, but this can be dangerous because it can damage your elbow joints. Make sure the inside creases of your elbows face one another.

2. **Pull your buttocks toward your feet and your knees toward your belly (see Figure 11-5a).**

   This is the starting position. You're squatting, except your knees are deeply bent. Feel your belly touching your thighs.

3. **Exhaling to a count of four, push your body up with your left leg as you lift your right leg toward the ceiling (see Figure 11-5b).**

   Keep both legs straight, if you can. Don't swing your back leg — press both legs firmly as you would the brakes in a car to come to a full stop. Look through your straightened arms at your left knee and shin.

   You can remove the leg weights or wear lighter weights if lifting your leg proves too difficult.

4. **Inhaling to a count of four, lower your right leg and return both legs to the starting position (see Figure 11-5a).**

   Look forward again as you squat.

Repeat this exercise six to eight times on each leg, take a rest, and then do six to eight more repetitions on each leg.

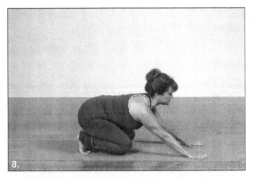

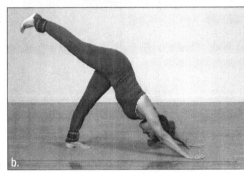

Figure 11-5: "Beep beep" your way to stronger abs and legs with the Road Runner.

The Side Bow

The Side Bow is an excellent exercise for people with unstable hips and pelvises — especially women — because it loosens and relaxes the front of your body, your hips, and your pelvis and stabilizes and strengthens those areas as well. The exercise also stretches your spine and works your quadriceps, buttocks, and abdominal muscles.

Strap on your ankle weights and follow these steps:

1. **Lie on your right side with your legs extended, resting on your right forearm for support.**

2. **Bend your left knee to a 45-degree angle, with your foot behind your buttocks (see Figure 11-6a).**

   This is the starting position. Keep your hips squared; don't shrug your shoulders or let your upper shoulder roll forward. Make sure your right hand stays on the floor for support.

3. **Exhaling to a count of four, press your left foot away from your body in a slow-motion donkey kick (see Figure 11-6b).**

   Push backward as hard as you can with your thigh and hip, not your knee. Feel your leg muscles working as you move.

   If you have too much trouble pushing, try doing this exercise without ankle weights.

4. **Inhaling to a count of four, return to the starting position (see Figure 11-6a).**

To get a good stretch when you're finished with the exercise, reach back and grasp the leg you just worked out with your hand. This stretches out your back and the quadriceps muscles of your leg.

Repeat this exercise six to eight times with each leg, take a rest, and then do six to eight more repetitions with each leg.

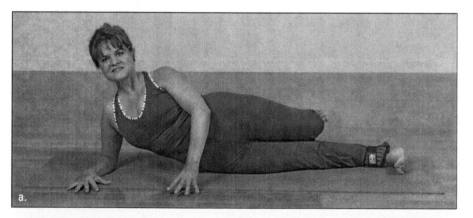

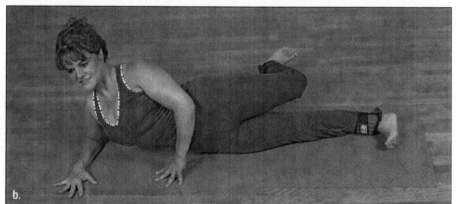

Figure 11-6:
The aim of the Side Bow is to work your buttocks.

The Horse

The Horse is based on a traditional yoga pose called the cobra. It's harder than it looks; then again, so is riding a horse! The exercise works your buttocks and the muscles of your abdomen, as well as muscles you may not even know about yet. It also massages your intestines and reproductive organs.

Strap on your ankle weights for the Horse and follow these steps:

1. **Lie on your belly with your elbows bent and on the ground under your shoulders and your hands grasping your arms right above the elbows (see Figure 11-7a).**

   Look downward, and grasp your arms like Mr. Clean (baby boomers, at least, will know who he is).

2. **Round your shoulders, lift your belly, round your back, and lower your forehead onto the top of your arms (see Figure 11-7b).**

   This is the starting position. Push into the floor with your elbows.

   You should draw your belly and tailbone down as you squeeze your perineum and buttocks. The *perineum* is the area between the anus and vagina in women and the anus and testicles in men. As you pull your belly in, feel the pose squeezing and massaging the organs behind your belly. Squeeze and engage these interior muscles throughout this exercise.

3. **Inhaling to a count of four, lift your right leg 6 inches off the floor (see Figure 11-7c).**

   In this position, you support some of your weight with your pubic bone. Make sure you keep your right leg straight as you lift.

   If you have trouble lifting your leg, tuck your belly in farther.

4. **Exhaling to a count of four, lower your right leg to the starting position (see Figure 11-7b).**

Take slow, full breaths throughout the exercise. You can't breathe deeply in the position you're in, but you can breathe consciously and mindfully.

You can do this exercise without the ankle weights and without lifting your leg. You still benefit your back and chest, and the exercise helps you develop a deeper and more rhythmic breathing pattern.

Do this exercise six to eight times with each leg, take a rest, and then do six to eight more repetitions with each leg.

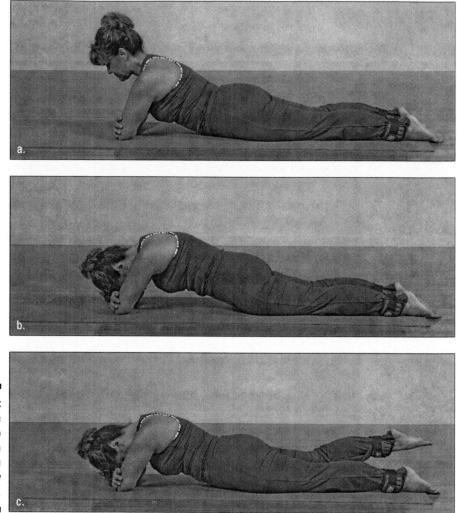

Figure 11-7:
The Horse
leads you to
soreness in
muscles you
didn't know
about.

The Ball

The Ball is a squeeze-and-soak exercise (it massages your internal organs)
that tucks you deep into the core of your body, and in doing so exercises
many different muscles. The exercise tones and conditions your neck, legs,
and abdominal muscles, and you develop balance, coordination, rhythm, and
timing.

You need your ankle weights for this exercise. When you're ready, follow these steps:

1. **Lie on your back with your head lifted, your knees bent and pulled toward your nose, and your fingers interlaced behind your knees (see Figure 11-8a).**

   This is the starting position. Look between your knees.

   If you can't interlace your fingers behind your knees, you can grasp the back of a leg with each hand.

2. **Inhaling to a count of four, simultaneously straighten your legs, lift them toward the ceiling, and lower your head to the floor (see Figure 11-8b).**

   Don't shrug your shoulders or tense your neck. Remember to draw your belly in; your belly muscles do some of the work of straightening and lifting your legs. Make sure your hands stay in contact with your knees, but don't pull your legs with your hands and arms.

   You can lift your legs halfway if you aren't flexible enough to straighten them.

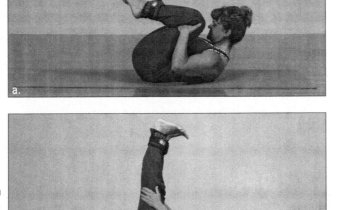

Figure 11-8: Have a ball by squeezing your torso.

3. **Exhaling to a count of four, lower and bend your legs and lift your head to return to the starting position (see Figure 11-8a).**

   Be careful not to roll your body. Stay in control. Let your four-count breathing guide you as you slowly lower your legs and return to the starting position.

Repeat this exercise six to eight times, take a rest, and then do six to eight more repetitions.

The Press

The Press is an exercise that borrows from weightlifting and from yoga. Your arms get the same workout you get from a bench press (without all the grunting you hear in a gym), and you get the benefits of a yogic leg raise. The exercise develops stamina and endurance, power, and strength; opens your groin; and stretches your hamstrings.

Grab your hand weights and ankle weights to do the Press. When you're ready, follow these steps:

1. **Holding the hand weights, lie on your back with your knees bent and feet off the ground and your elbows bent and to the side of your shoulders (see Figure 11-9a).**

   This is the starting position. Raise your forearms above your shoulders, and raise your legs above your hips. You look like an upside-down table. The bottoms of your feet should be perpendicular to the ceiling.

2. **Exhaling to a count of four, simultaneously lift your head, hands, and feet toward the ceiling (see Figure 11-9b).**

   Imagine that you're pushing a heavy object away from your body with your arms and legs. Engage your belly muscles as you lift.

3. **Inhaling to a count of four, return to the starting position (see Figure 11-9a).**

   Keep your shoulders squared. Don't drop the weights; gently lower them.

Repeat this exercise six to eight times, take a rest, and then do six to eight more repetitions.

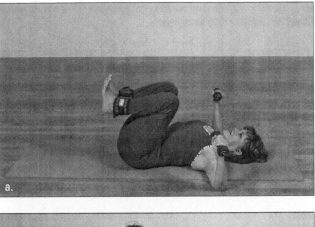

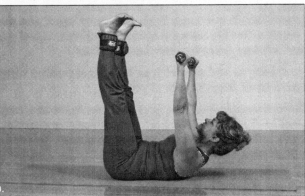

Figure 11-9:
The Press is a bench press and leg press rolled into one.

The Straddle

The Straddle can improve your health and physical performance whether you like to walk around the block or enjoy mountain climbing. The exercise loosens and expands the range of motion in your pelvis and legs, opens your groin, and conditions and tones your back. The pose also builds abdominal strength and works your biceps. The Straddle is tough, but stay with it. The benefits it gives your groin help in both walking and climbing.

Throughout this exercise, don't cave in or round your back or shoulders. Doing so may strain your back.

You need both hand weights and ankle weights for this exercise. After you're locked and loaded, follow these steps:

1. **Sit on your buttocks with your legs spread apart and the ankle weights resting on your inner thighs (see Figure 11-10a).**

   Putting weights on your inner thighs helps anchor your hips. The hand weights can rest on the floor behind you; don't worry about them just yet. The tips of your toes should be facing the ceiling.

   If you happen to be flexible, you may be tempted to open your legs too wide, but be careful. You can injure yourself during the weightlifting part of this exercise if your legs are too far apart.

2. **Roll the fleshy part of each buttock and thigh out from under you.**

   To do this, pull your belly in, lean to one side, reach around your hip, grasp your buttock and inner thigh with your hand, and move the flesh to the outside. Do this for each buttock. You should feel your "sit bones" and your tailbone pressing down into the floor.

   Draw your belly in and up and your tailbone down for support, and flex and press into all four corners of your feet.

   If you have discomfort in your back and you begin to slouch your shoulders, your back muscles may not be ready for this exercise. Just move your legs a little closer and find your natural seat. You can also tuck one foot in or sit on a rolled-up mat or towel.

3. **Pick up the hand weights and curl them so that your triceps are parallel with your shoulders (see Figure 11-10b).**

   This is the starting position.

4. **Inhaling to a count of four, extend your arms to form a T position with your head and torso (see Figure 11-10c).**

   Align your shoulders over your hips. Your palms should be facing upward.

5. **Exhaling to a count of four, lift the weights back to the starting position (see Figure 11-10b).**

Repeat this exercise six to eight times, take a rest, and then do six to eight more repetitions.

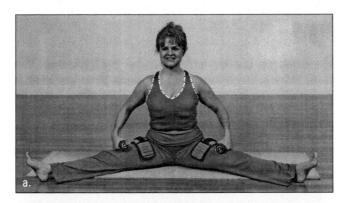

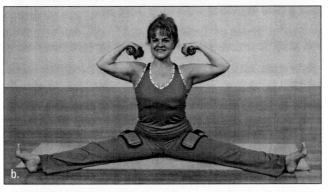

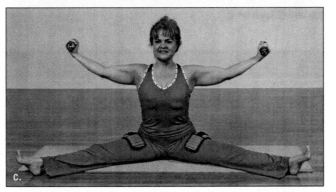

Figure 11-10:
The Straddle opens and strengthens your groin and pelvis.

The Recharge

The Recharge helps you unwind and relax after the Endurance Workout. The exercise should release the tension and fatigue in your forehead and brow. The breathing portion of the exercise benefits your mind, body, and spirit.

Grab your ankle weights and follow these steps:

1. **Sit with your legs crossed and your ankles beside your heels, and place the ankle weights on your thighs.**

   Adding the weights helps sink your thighs into the floor.

2. **Rub your palms together until they heat up.**

   Perhaps you've heard of "healing hands?" Well, you've got a pair of them with you at all times. Use the warmth of your own two hands to heal.

3. **Close your eyes, and gently cup your hands over your eyes (see Figure 11-11).**

   The idea is to block out light without putting pressure on your eyes. Let the warmth of your hands soften and release any tension in your forehead and brow. In traditional yoga, placing warm palms over the eyes is called *palming*.

4. **Take six to ten Complete Breaths.**

   A Complete Breath is a deep, relaxing breath. (For more on Complete Breaths, see Chapter 4.)

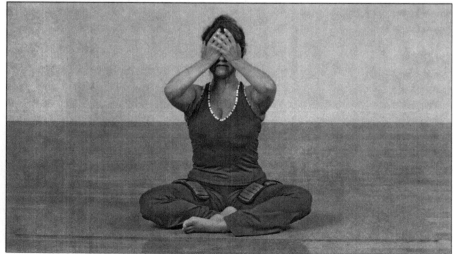

Figure 11-11:
Palming
your eyes
recharges
your
batteries.

Ending Meditation

After you finish the Endurance Workout, take a moment to engage in meditation. Meditation isn't about sitting still or forcing yourself to be quiet; it's about anchoring your consciousness into the present moment. You deepen your relationship to your breath in a calm and steady way. The common aim is to focus the scattered rays of your mind on a single point, like a laser beam of attention, in order to lead you to a state of self-realization. Chapter 6 describes several meditation techniques.

Chapter 12

Iron Abs: The Belly-Burner Workout

In This Chapter

▶ Strengthening the core muscles of your abdomen and back

▶ Shaping and toning your trunk

▶ Burning the fat from your belly

▶ Massaging and toning the organs of digestion and elimination

*E*verybody wants strong abdominal muscles, because having strong abs means having a flatter, trimmer stomach. Many people don't know it, but strong abdominal and back muscles are as important for your overall good health as for your good looks. The abdominal center is the mother of all movement because movement from this core area empowers all other movement, including that of the head, legs, and arms. Strong abs support the integrity of many muscle groups that are necessary for having a healthy back, which makes strong abs necessary for good posture. Having a healthy back and abs go hand in hand — like love and marriage or cookies and milk, you can't have one without the other.

In the Belly-Burner Workout, you notice immediately that the moves are initiated from the abdominal core of your body, and you can tell right away how strong or weak you are in this area. The exercises focus on the abdominal core and help you carve out muscle tone and build stability. They also improve circulation and massage and tone the organs of digestion and elimination.

If your goal is to shrink your belly area, you've come to the right place. If you do them for 20 to 30 minutes every other day and eat less, the Belly-Burner exercises will help immensely. This workout gets you juiced up and running like a well-tuned and efficient energy-burning machine.

Throughout this workout, you should practice the Ocean Breath. Chapter 4 explains this and several other yoga breaths.

The Cow to Cat

The Cow to Cat (call it the Curl and Crunch if you like) works your abdominal muscles much like a stomach crunch; it's soothing to your neck and back; it stretches and strengthens your spine; and it works your legs and buttocks. Why the unusual name? Because in the first part of the exercise, you stretch your chest and make it look like the big, broad face of a cow. In the second part, when you round your back, you look like a Halloween cat.

Wear your ankle weights for this exercise. When you're ready, follow these steps:

1. **Start on all fours with your knees directly under your hips and your wrists directly under your shoulders.**

   Make sure your fingers are spread wide for support and balance. You look like a table in this position.

2. **Inhaling to a count of four, lower your belly down as you move your back one vertebra at a time into a full stretch with your chin up (see Figure 12-1a).**

   This is the cow position. Keep your hips parallel during this step (and throughout this exercise).

3. **Exhaling to a count of four, round your back and tuck in your chin as you lift your right knee toward your chest (see Figure 12-1b).**

   This, the cat position, is the starting position. Look down into your navel or at your knee.

   Move your tailbone down and pull your belly in and up as you do this portion of the exercise.

4. **Inhaling to a count of four, lift your right leg directly behind you as you raise your chin (see Figure 12-1c).**

   Spread your toes wide, and lift your leg to hip level. Imagine that you're pressing your foot into a wall. Don't kick or swing your leg; move it slowly to work the muscles of your buttocks. Keep your toes pointed toward the ground if you can.

   Feel your back arch as you do this part of the exercise.

5. **Exhaling to a count of four, return to the starting position (see Figure 12-1b).**

   Be careful not to drop your head; lower it slowly into your chest. Concentrate on your lungs emptying and your belly squeezing as you exhale.

The stretching and contracting of your abdominal muscles helps you tone and shape them.

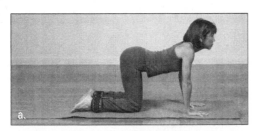

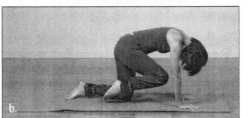

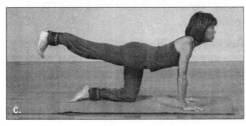

Figure 12-1:
Who said turning a cow into a cat would be easy on your abs and back?

Repeat this exercise six to eight times with each leg, take a rest, and then do six to eight more repetitions with each leg.

The Flying Locust

The Flying Locust is a weighted variation of a classic yoga pose that allows you to pretend you're in flight. The exercise strengthens and tones the front and back of your body. It also strengthens your shoulders, arms, chest, legs, and buttocks. You support your body weight with your abdominal muscles in the process, which is why it works as a big-time belly buster.

The Flying Locust is a difficult exercise. To do it right, you need to pay attention each moment during the exercise. If any part of your back feels uncomfortable, you can do this exercise with light hand weights or with no weights at all until you get strong enough.

You need both ankle and hand weights for this exercise. When you're ready, follow these steps:

1. **Lie flat on your belly with your forehead touching the floor, your arms spread in a T position, and your hands holding the hand weights palms-down (see Figure 12-2a).**

   This is the starting position.

2. **Inhaling to a count of four, lift your arms, your legs, and your chin straight up off the ground (see Figure 12-2b).**

   Without jerking your body or throwing your head back, try to lift up at the same rate and to the same height. As you do this, notice your shoulders moving away from your ears and your shoulder blades moving toward each other. Pull your belly in and up and your tailbone down as you lift. Keep your legs directly behind you.

   You should feel your abdominal muscles tighten in this position. The weight of your body is falling on these muscles, and they must stay engaged to support your body.

   It helps to imagine that someone is pressing on the back of your head and that you have to hold your head up. Lifting your head properly helps get your shoulders and arms up.

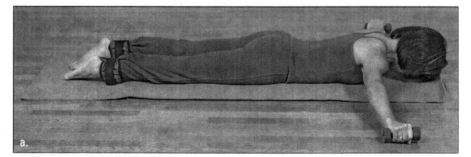

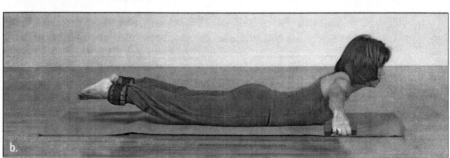

Figure 12-2: Imagine the buzzing of insects as you fly through this exercise.

3. **Exhaling to a count of four, slowly lower your arms, legs, and chin to the starting position (see Figure 12-2a).**

   Don't drop your limbs; lower them in time to your breathing.

If you try the Flying Locust and have trouble lifting the weights from the T position, try keeping your hands alongside your hips without the weights.

Repeat this exercise six to eight times, pause to rest, and then do six to eight more repetitions.

The Locust

The Locust offers many of the same benefits as the Flying Locust (see the previous exercise in this workout). It develops your shoulders, chest, arms, legs, back, buttocks, and abdominal muscles. Instead of working all four limbs at the same time, however, you work only two — an opposite arm and leg. For this reason, the Locust develops cross-coordination and fires the nerve pathways of your brain.

If the Locust proves too difficult at first, use lighter weights, or do the exercise without weights until you develop your strength.

Pick up one hand weight and strap on both ankle weights for this exercise. When you're ready, follow these steps:

1. **Lie flat on your belly with your forehead resting on your right forearm and your left arm extended vertically, holding the hand weight palm-down (see Figure 12-3a).**

   This, the starting position, is sometimes called the skydiving position. Draw your belly in and up and your tailbone down for support.

2. **Inhaling to a count of four, lift your right leg, your left arm, and your shoulders and head (see Figure 12-3b).**

   In other words, lift your opposite arm and leg as you lift from the shoulders up. Rise to a position that works your muscles but doesn't strain them. Gently but firmly press down on your forearm to help lift your head and shoulders.

   You can keep your head down in a neutral position or lift your head when you lift your arm and leg; the choice is yours. If you want to lift your head, keep your ear in proximity to the lifting arm, and be careful not to toss your head — lift it slowly.

3. **Exhaling to a count of four, lower your arm, leg, shoulders, and head to the starting position (see Figure 12-3a).**

Feel the strain in your abdominal muscles as you slowly work your opposite limbs.

Repeat this exercise six to eight times with each arm-leg combination, pause to rest, and then do six to eight more repetitions with each arm-leg combo.

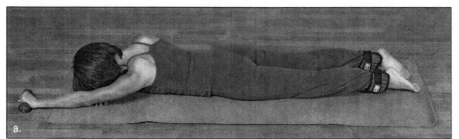

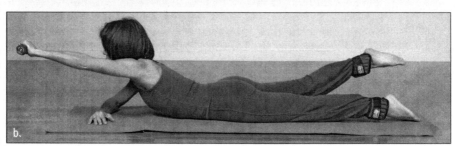

Figure 12-3:
The Locust works your core muscles and focuses on your coordination and balance.

The Love Handler

As its name implies, the Love Handler is designed to shrink the size of your love handles — the excess weight around your waistline. Many people accumulate fat in this area as a result of stress. This gentle, side-bending exercise stretches and tones your *obliques* and the *rectus abdominis* — Latin for "love handles." The exercise not only works the aforementioned Latin muscles, but also helps to relieve stress when you stretch and breathe deeply.

You need one hand weight and both ankle weights for this exercise. When you're ready, follow these steps:

1. **Sit on your buttocks with your right leg extended, your left hand gently pressing down into the floor, your left foot tucked next to your right thigh, and the hand weight held at hip position in your right hand (see Figure 12-4a).**

This is the starting position — a position similar to that of a hurdler. Try to sit deep into your buttock on the bent-knee side to anchor you and enable you to stretch farther. The ankle weights act as anchors for your body during the exercise.

Make sure your spine is erect, your belly is tucked in, and your tailbone is pointing down. Look straight ahead, with your chin neither raised nor lowered.

2. **Inhaling to a count of four, arc the hand weight over your body as you turn your head to the left and look down toward your fingertips (see Figure 12-4b).**

   As you do this, lean to the left. Don't throw the weight — lift it carefully. As you lift, rotate the weight in your hand. Feel the right side of your body — especially your love handle — stretching. Use your left hand for support as you look over your left shoulder.

3. **Exhaling to a count of four, return the hand weight and your body to the starting position (see Figure 12-4a).**

   Feel the muscle on the side of your body draw you back to the starting position.

This is a terrific lateral — that is, side-bending — stretch. Be careful not to lean forward or feel as if you're falling backward during this exercise. If you do, you'll lose the benefits of stretching your love handles.

Repeat this exercise six to eight times on each side of your body, take a rest, and then do six to eight more repetitions on each side.

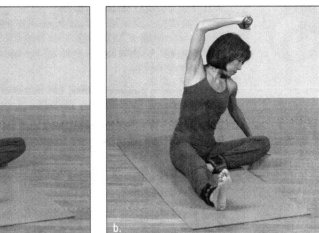

Figure 12-4:
The Love Handler reduces the size of your infamous love handles.

The Staff

The Staff is a weighted version of the traditional yoga pose of uprightness. The exercise builds a strong spine and back. The weights appear to exercise the muscles of your back and shoulders, which they do, but the main object of the Staff is to exercise your abdominal muscles. A secondary benefit is the work you do on your quads and hamstrings.

Don't collapse your spine as you do this exercise (in other words, don't slump). If you don't keep your spine erect and your elbows square, you won't work your abdominal muscles.

You need both hand weights and ankle weights for this exercise. When you're ready, follow these steps:

1. **Sit on your buttocks with your legs straight in front of you, and roll the fleshy part of each buttock and thigh out from under your body.**

   Pull your belly in, lean to one side, reach around your hip, grasp your buttock and inner thigh with your hand, and move the flesh to the outside. Do this for each buttock. After you finish, you'll feel as if your "sit bones" are rooted downward a little bit more toward the floor. You'll also be able to draw your belly in and work your abdominal muscles more deeply.

2. **Grab the hand weights and bend your arms, holding the weights at ear level with your palms facing forward (see Figure 12-5a).**

   This is the starting position. Don't shrug your shoulders; look straight ahead throughout the exercise.

   If sitting upright while holding the weights is too uncomfortable for you, try placing a rolled-up blanket under your buttocks to encourage your pelvis to release. This way, you feel the natural curve of your lumbar spine again, which helps you sit up taller and straighter. You can also bend your knees.

3. **Inhaling to a count of four, lift the weights straight up so your arms are extended (see Figure 12-5b).**

   This action is what weightlifters call an *overhead press*. Engage your feet, flexing into all four corners to encourage you to tighten your abdominal muscles.

4. **Exhaling to a count of four, lower your arms to the starting position (see Figure 12-5a).**

   Feel your shoulder blades pulling down in rhythm to your breathing. As you slowly lower the weights, feel yourself working against the weight for resistance. This action is what weightlifters call a *back lat pulldown*.

Focus on your belly as you lift and lower the weights; your belly muscles support your back and spine.

Repeat this exercise six to eight times, pause to rest, and then do six to eight more repetitions.

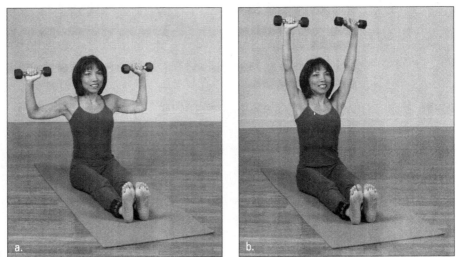

Figure 12-5:
The Staff works to build a strong spine and back.

The Burning Boat

The Burning Boat really works the muscles of your belly, like rowing without paddles. Because you exercise with only your buttocks touching the ground, you make your muscles burn and you build endurance and stamina. In the yogic system, fire represents purification, change, and renewal. Be sure to use Ocean Breaths (see Chapter 4) in this workout because they oxygenate the fire and really heat things up.

You need both hand weights and ankle weights for this exercise. When you're ready, follow these steps.

1. **Sit on your buttocks with your knees bent and feet flat on the floor, and hold the weights in your hands with your palms facing forward (see Figure 12-6a).**

    Pull your belly in, and lift your spine.

2. **Lean back slightly, lift your feet from the floor, and tuck your knees into your chest (see Figure 12-6b).**

    This is the starting position. Concentrate on finding a point of balance.

    If you have a lower back injury, lift one leg at a time rather than both legs. If you still feel uncomfortable, move on to the next exercise.

If your abdominal muscles are strong enough, you can try doing this exercise with your legs straight, not bent.

3. **Exhaling to a count of four, lift the hand weights to perform a bicep curl (see Figure 12-6c).**

Keep your shoulders squared to place the work directly on your bicep muscles.

Be careful not to drop the weights. Let the rhythm of your breathing guide your motion.

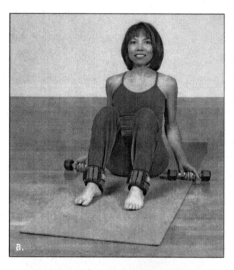
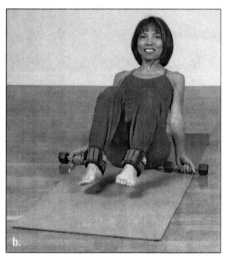
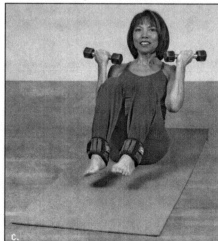

Figure 12-6: The Burning Boat requires oodles of strength and abdominal fortitude.

4. **Inhaling to a count of four, lower the hand weights to the starting position (see Figure 12-6b).**

Don't hold your breath during this exercise. Focus on your breathing, and try to relax (yeah, right!).

If doing this exercise with weights is too difficult at first, try it without the weights or with light weights until you become strong enough.

Repeat this exercise six to eight times, take a rest, and then do six to eight more repetitions.

The Archer

The aim of the Archer is to work the lower abdominal muscles that often get ignored in traditional upper-ab building sit-ups. Imagine you're squeezing — really squeezing — the juice from an orange in your lower belly as you do this exercise.

You need only your ankle weights for the Archer. Lock, load, and follow these steps:

1. **Lie on your back with your right leg extended, your left leg bent toward your chest, and your fingers interlaced about 2 inches below your left knee (see Figure 12-7a).**

   This is the starting position. Keep your arms straight, and press your knee into your hands.

2. **Exhaling to a count of four, lift your head and right leg off the ground as you continue to hold your left knee (see Figure 12-7b).**

   Lift with your lower belly muscles; don't pull on your knee or leg to lift your body. Press your knee powerfully into your hands as you feel your lower abdominal muscles and back working. See how going from a fully relaxed to a fully flexed position really challenges your abdominal muscles.

3. **Inhaling to a count of four, lower your head and right leg to return to the starting position (see Figure 12-7a).**

Keep your feet engaged throughout this exercise to help you work your abdominal muscles. By focusing on your breathing, you can do this exercise slowly and consciously without tugging on your leg or jerking your back.

Repeat this exercise six to eight times with each leg, take a rest, and then do six to eight more repetitions with each leg.

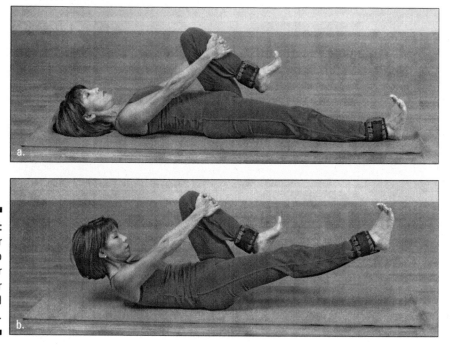

Figure 12-7:
The Archer
aims to
sculpt your
lower
abdominal
muscles.

The Pearl

The Pearl works your abdominal muscles and stretches out your spine while making your legs and arms stronger. You have to concentrate and stay in the moment to perfect this exercise, which strengthens your mind as well as the muscles of your body. The Pearl is also a squeeze-and-soak exercise that massages your intestines and other internal organs. You start by opening up like an oyster, and then you pull tight like a pearl; the treasure is within you!

You need both hand and ankle weights for this exercise. When you're ready, follow these steps:

1. **Lie on your back with your arms extended above your head, your palms facing upward while holding the hand weights, and your legs straight (see Figure 12-8a).**

   This is the starting position.

2. **Exhaling to a count of four, slowly move your arms toward the ceiling and back down toward your sides in a half-circle while you bend your knees into your chest and lift your forehead toward your knees (see Figure 12-8b).**

Curl your back one vertebra at a time so your head and neck lift last. Feel your belly squeezing and burning.

Your arms should be in a position beside your hips a few inches above the floor as you pull them forward like a round pearl.

Instead of raising your legs to your chest from an extended position, you can try this exercise with bent knees and your feet on the floor. It still poses a challenge, but because you don't lift as much body weight, it isn't as hard.

3. **Inhaling to a count of four, slowly return to the starting position (see Figure 12-8a).**

   Feel your abdominal muscles working and burning as you uncrunch.

Controlled action is the key to success in this exercise. Move slowly and consciously — especially when you lower your arms behind your head.

Repeat this exercise six to eight times, pause to rest, and then do six to eight more repetitions.

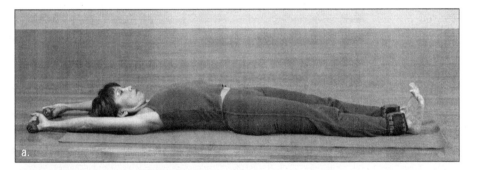

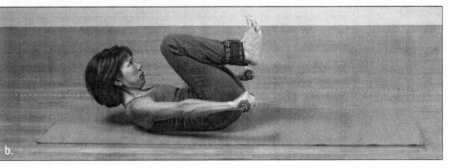

Figure 12-8: Crunch deep into your body to create the pearl within.

The Belly Crunch

The Belly Crunch does exactly what it says — it crunches your abdominal muscles in a very big yoga-with-weights way. This exercise works your waist-line as well as your deep abdominal muscles. The crossover action in this exercise helps to strengthen and tone your back and waistline even more. As long as you perform the movements slowly without throwing your body, you'll really feel your abdominal muscles working. Crunch that belly a few times and watch it start to flatten out as your waistline takes shape.

If you have a neck injury, don't attempt this exercise. It may place too much strain on your neck, a major contributor of support for your body in this exercise. (In Chapter 14, you find some great exercises and suggestions for strengthening your back and neck.)

Grab your hand weights and strap on your ankle weights for this exercise. When you're ready, follow these steps:

1. **Lie on your back with your knees tucked into your chest and your bent elbows in the scarecrow position (see Figure 12-9a).**

   This is the starting position.

   In the scarecrow position, you stretch your arms out wide at shoulder level and bend your elbows at 90-degree angles. Make sure an equal distance lies between your hands and head and your elbows and shoulders.

2. **Exhaling to a count of four, lift your head, touch your left elbow to your right knee, and extend your left leg into the air (see Figure 12-9b).**

   Keep your abdominals engaged at all times, and press through your feet to feel stronger in your belly muscles.

   If lifting your head is too much trouble or your neck gets too tired, keep your head on the floor. You can also do this exercise without ankle or hand weights.

3. **Inhaling to a count of four, bring your left leg back into your chest, cross your right elbow to your left knee, and extend your right leg into the air.**

   Don't bring your head down as you do this.

4. **Exhaling to a count of four, tuck both knees back into your chest and lie back into the starting position (see Figure 12-9a).**

Draw your belly down and in as you lift, and twist the trunk of your body as you touch your elbows to your knees. As you twist, imagine that you're wringing out a dishrag. And remember to keep moving between legs. Although this is a slow and controlled exercise, your momentum will carry you along.

Do this exercise six to eight times with each leg and elbow combination, pause to rest, and then do another six to eight repetitions with each leg and elbow combo.

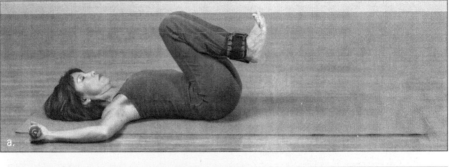

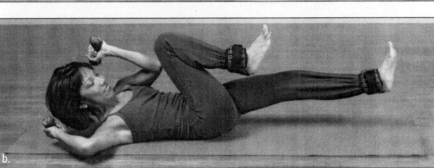

Figure 12-9:
The Belly Crunch focuses on your abdominal muscles.

The Belly Dancer

You deserve a relaxing exercise if you've come this far. Although belly dancing doesn't sound relaxing, the Belly Dancer gives you an opportunity to loosen up and have some fun. The exercise strengthens your pelvic girdle as it loosens and removes the tension from your spine. This relaxing and soothing exercise closes out your Belly-Burner Workout, setting you up for a belly full of laughter.

You need one ankle weight and both hand weights for this exercise. When you're ready, follow these steps:

1. **Lie on your back with your knees bent, your feet on the floor, the ankle weight placed on your belly, and your arms at your sides, holding the hand weights palms-down.**

   This is the starting position. The added weight on your belly brings your attention to this area of your body.

2. **Lift your buttocks 4 to 6 inches from the floor as you tilt your tailbone toward your navel (see Figure 12-10).**

   Sculpt your belly in and up.

3. **Gently sway your hips like a pendulum from side to side.**

   Feel your spine lengthening and stretching as you make this soothing, rocking motion. Don't lift your hips any higher than you already have.

4. **Continue swaying your hips until you release the tension from your body.**

For fun at the end of the exercise, do a few figure-eight patterns in each direction, and then shimmy and wiggle for ten seconds to a minute. Enjoy the natural dance and rhythm of your movement!

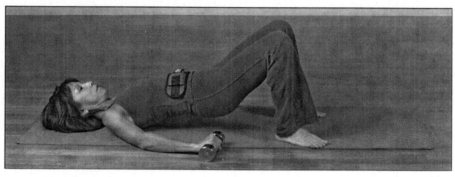

Figure 12-10: Make like a Belly Dancer as you relax your abs and back.

Ending Meditation

Before you leave the Belly-Burner Workout behind, we encourage you to take a moment to engage in meditation. You can quietly collect yourself and get ready for the next activity you want to do. Look to Chapter 6 to find a meditation technique that you enjoy.

Part III
Refining Your Technique

The 5th Wave   By Rich Tennant

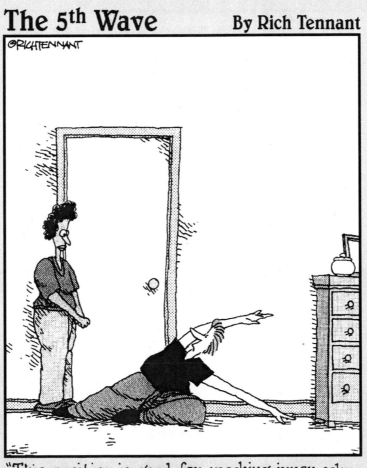

"This position is good for reaching inner calm, mental clarity, and things that roll behind the refrigerator."

In this part . . .

Part III is the heart of this book. It offers five yoga-with-weights workouts designed to energize, restore, strengthen, or tone different parts of your body.

Try the Energy Workout (Chapter 8) when your energy starts to wane and you need a boost. Hit up the Restorative Workout (Chapter 9) when you want to feel alert and wide awake. When you want to get stronger, the Strengthening Workout (Chapter 10) is for you, and when you want to increase your stamina, go to the Endurance Workout (Chapter 11). Are your pants too tight? Better try the Belly-Burner Workout (Chapter 12). Good luck!

Chapter 13

Eating to Enhance Your Yoga-with-Weights Workout

For many years, Sherri's family ran health centers in San Francisco. One very popular center had a health-food store on the bottom floor; the upper floors were reserved for a gym, a yoga room, and a dance studio. Over the years, Sherri noticed that many of the visitors to the center either went to the top floors for yoga, bodybuilding, dance, or other forms of exercise or to the bottom floor to purchase health foods or to eat in the health-food restaurant. Not everyone visited both places, but the people who did really looked great. They radiated good health. The observations reinforced for Sherri that exercise and nutrition go hand in hand.

Doing yoga-with-weights exercises inspires you to want to feel your best and to tune in to your body's needs. Before you put anything in your mouth, you pause to make sure that it's really worth eating. Your energy and increased mental clarity feel good as a result of yoga with weights, and you don't want to lose that. As with any dynamic form of exercising, yoga with weights places demands on your body. To meet those demands, you need to put the right fuel into your body. You need to eat foods that give you the energy for exercising and building strong muscle and bone. You don't attempt to power a car with water. Similarly, you can't power your body — you can't get the energy you need to exercise — without eating the right foods.

This chapter isn't a diet book in miniature. It doesn't tell you what to eat and what not to eat. It does, however, offer basic and simple suggestions to help you find good health and to help you get the energy you need to do yoga-with-weights workouts.

Listening to the Wisdom of Your Body

One of the keys to improving your diet is to be aware of what your body tells you to eat. You were born with an inner awareness that steers you to foods that make you feel your best. Try to tap into this awareness. What you eat and how you take care of yourself influence your energy level, your mood, your frame of mind, and your temperament. Ask yourself these questions: "What did I eat for my last meal? Have I had a snack recently? How do I feel right now? Am I thirsty?" What you consume contributes to how you feel right now.

As the saying goes, you are what you eat. Everyone understands that drugs and medicines have direct effects on the body, but few people stop to consider what effect foods have. Eating sugary foods, for example, gives most people an energy rush. These foods cause your blood-sugar (or glucose) level to spike for a short period of time, which feels good. You feel like you have more energy, and you may even feel happier for a little while. But then you experience a rapid drop in blood-sugar that leaves you feeling drained of energy. Being aware of your body's responses to different foods can direct you to foods that bring energy, health, and vitality.

Think of the food you eat as medicine — it provides vitamins and minerals that are essential not only for good health, but also for strong muscles and a sound mind.

No two people are the same, which is why we don't recommend the same diet for everyone. Writes Dr. Elson Haas, author of *The New Detox Diet Book: Staying Healthy with Nutrition* (Celestial Arts) and *Vitamins For Dummies* (Wiley), "Our diet, or best eating program, is an individual exploration and there is no one right diet for everyone. Our heritage, seasonal and local environment, activity level, digestion and health state all influence what makes up our best diet. That's why the personal attunement process is so crucial."

To eat nutritiously, you don't have to follow a strict diet like it's the letter of the law or even follow someone else's rules about what constitutes a good diet. You can follow what we like to call the *85–15 percent principal:* Eat at least 85 percent of the time from the group of healthy whole and organic foods; the other 15 percent of your diet is for the occasional splurge or treat, a big dinner party, or a grand fiesta. Having a base of good, wholesome foods gives your body the foundation it needs to be healthy enough to deal with the occasional treat or splurge.

Starting an exercise program and changing your diet all at once can seem like an overwhelming proposition. If you're unsure how to change your diet, and you don't know where to start, we encourage you to seek help. Consult a credentialed expert in nutrition. Find out from an expert what diet is best for you. Get help in tracking your responses to different kinds of food and different food groups.

Improving Your Diet through Yoga with Weights

When you do yoga-with-weights exercises, you explore your body. You discover how to relax certain muscles and flex others; you retrace the pathways of your nerves and find out how different muscle groups work in consort when you balance; you feel your breath bring life-giving oxygen to your body; and you discover many new feelings and sensations.

It may seem far-fetched, but yoga with weights, an exercise program, can actually improve your diet. If the yoga-with-weights program has one theme, it's this: Listen to your body so you hear what it's trying to tell you. Yoga with weights helps you get in touch with your body. You gain not only an awareness of how your body reacts to the movements you make with the weights, but also calm and inner composure, which can be helpful in preventing nervous eating. You no longer experience the unnatural hunger spasms caused by anxiety because your thoughts are more in tune with the health needs of your body.

We encourage you to understand where your stress or fatigue comes from and how it affects your eating. If your exercise goal is to lose weight, you can lose it without having to count calories or measure food portions. You lose it because losing weight isn't an objective in and of itself; it's a side effect of the feeling of well-being, the increased movement, and the exercise you get from practicing yoga with weights.

If you concentrate on the principles of yoga with weights and adhere to your goals, when you're hungry and you need to eat more, you'll make better choices about what to eat. It may take some time, but eventually you'll begin to select from foods that give you the energy to do the exercises without the excess calories. You'll notice a lighter feeling overall because your body doesn't have to work as hard to digest food or recover from having eaten processed, fat-laden, unnatural food. You'll have the firsthand experience and the confidence in yourself to know when you can eat with abundance from the right sources. Your yoga-with-weights self-awareness training can help guide you to the right foods.

Following Guidelines for Healthy Eating

We encourage you to eat a healthy diet of fresh foods, fruits, vegetables, protein, whole grains, and some dairy products (if you tolerate them well). These foods provide energy, and your body can absorb and make use of them easily. In some quarters, this natural way of eating is known as the *whole-food diet*. Discover how good you can feel from eating fresh and healthy foods in their more natural, whole-food state.

Food is the guardian of your health and the source of energy in your daily life. Some of the foods we discuss in this chapter aren't a part of most diets, but most people haven't taken up the beneficial yoga-with-weights lifestyle that you have. These foods are powerful, simple, and effective in supporting good health.

Discovering the value of whole foods

Whole foods are natural foods that come to us as nature made them. They haven't been altered by chemical processes, and they don't have preservatives or additives that prolong their shelf lives or make them taste better. These foods often contain more vitamins, minerals, fiber, complex carbohydrates, and essential fatty acids than processed foods.

How do you tell whole foods from other foods? Generally speaking, whole foods come to you as nature made them. For example, raw and steamed vegetables and fresh fruits are whole foods. Whole wheat, whole grains (brown rice, kasha, millet, and so on), nuts, seeds, legumes (lentils, peas, beans), eggs, fish, lean meats, poultry, and unrefined oils are other examples. Refined foods that you want to steer clear of include white sugar, white rice, and white flour. Often, you're still hungry after you eat refined food. You crave food sooner because you haven't been properly nourished, so you eat more. That means bad news for your yoga-with-weights workout. Bye-bye motivation and energy, hello couch and nap.

Often, but not exclusively, whole foods are grown by using organic or sustainable-farming methods. In a way, they're a step back to the good old days, when people grew their own food and harvested on their own. They ate foods local to their areas and the places where they were born. People used to limit their diets to foods that were in season. They ate fresh food because they had to — they had no refrigerators.

Whole foods are pure and unrefined. They have a higher nutritional density, and they present nutrients to your body in such a way that your body can recognize them, absorb them, and take full advantage of their nutritional power by supplying you with the energy you need to do your yoga-with-weights workouts. When you eat whole foods and include plenty of fresh fruits and vegetables as the basis of your diet, you don't have to eat as much to get the vitamins and minerals you need.

A great place to find whole foods is your local farmer's market. Lucky for you, farmer's markets are popping up everywhere in cities and towns. These markets provide wonderful fresh and seasonal foods that, for the most part, are grown locally. Farmer's markets often have live music to shop by and plenty of people worth watching. You can have a feast for your eyes and palate.

Including dairy products in your diet

Dairy products, if you can tolerate them, are great sources of calcium — which is necessary for strong bones and teeth — vitamin D, and protein. Protein, especially, is good for yoga-with-weights practitioners because it's a great source of energy and it helps to maintain healthy muscle tissue. Calcium also helps support healthy bone density.

When you consume milk, cheese, and yogurt, do so in moderation, or consume the low-fat and nonfat varieties of dairy products. Many dairy products are high in saturated fats, and saturated fat is a risk factor for heart disease; in women, it may also be a risk factor in breast and ovarian cancer. Try to purchase eggs (from free-range hens) that are high in omega-3 fatty acids. Studies show that omega-3 fatty acids are helpful against high blood pressure and heart disease.

High-quality yogurt and kefir are helpful additions to your diet. These cultured foods contain friendly bacteria — *Lactobacillus acidophillus, Lactobacillus bulgaricus,* and others — that make it harder for unfriendly bacteria to live in your gut. You can spot a high-quality yogurt because its label tells you that it contains "live bacteria cultures." Don't be shy about eating goat and sheep's milk products; they're rich in calcium and very good for your health.

Supplying your body with proteins

To build muscles for your yoga-with-weights workouts, you need protein and the amino acids from which protein is made. Like bricks to a house, proteins are your body's basic building materials. Your body uses protein to build new cells and tissue and to create hormones, enzymes, and antibodies. When you eat protein, your body breaks it down into amino acids.

The best suppliers of protein are animal sources. Milk, eggs, chicken, beef, and fish are called *complete proteins* because they supply all the essential amino acids. Fruits and vegetables are called *incomplete proteins* because they don't supply all the essential amino acids.

Your protein needs are different from the person working out next to you in the gym; some people even have trouble absorbing proteins. If your digestive system can't absorb protein, the undigested protein simply passes through your digestive tract without being absorbed and used by your body. Protein sources that are high in fiber, for example, are harder to digest. Make sure you can absorb the protein from food and that the protein meal contains all the essential amino acids.

How much protein is enough? How does a vegetarian combine foods to get enough protein? How much is too much? Take subjects of concern up with a physician or a qualified nutritionist. He or she can help you figure how much protein you need, given your body's needs and your lifestyle.

Tasty cooking with monounsaturated fat

If you're looking for a good source of monoun-saturated fat and don't want to give up a tasty diet, include olive oil in your diet. It's great for salads and works well in cooking. You shouldn't heat olive oil too high, however, and you should refrigerate it.

Many farmer's markets specialize in fresh oils; often, you can sample the oils before buying.

You can find a wide selection of flavors ranging from bitter to buttery to almost lemony. Cold-pressed, first-run, extra virgin olive oil is the best because it's unrefined. Try to buy the oil in small amounts, store it in dark or opaque bottles, and consume it while it's fresh — oils exposed to light may become rancid in no time.

Consuming healthy fats and essential fatty acids

"Fat" has become a bad word in American culture, but fats are nothing to be afraid of. Some fats, in fact, are important for a healthy diet and are good for you. Fat provides vitamins A, D, and E and plays an important role in the health of your bones, skin, and hair. Fats are also important for mineral absorption.

Of course, not all fat is created equal. Some fats are better than others, but generally they fall into these three categories:

- **Saturated fat:** You find these fats in animal and dairy products. They include butter, cheese, whole milk, ice cream, cream, and fatty meats. You can eat foods with saturated fats now and then, but not too often. These fats contain high levels of low-density lipoprotein (LDL), the "bad cholesterol," and they've been implicated in heart disease.

- **Monounsaturated fat:** These fats come from plant sources. They include olive, canola, and peanut oils; avocado; and nuts (almonds, pecans, peanuts, and cashews). Monounsaturated fat is high in calories, but it's excellent for your health because it lowers cholesterol levels in your blood and helps prevent heart disease.

- **Polyunsaturated fat:** This fat is useful against blood clotting, heart disease, and high blood pressure. Polyunsaturated fats go rancid quickly if you don't refrigerate them. The fats fall in two categories:

  - **Omega-3** essential fatty acid is found in free-range poultry and in eggs. Most people don't get enough healthy Omega-3 in their diets. The best sources of this fat are free-range eggs and cold-water ocean fish such as salmon, tuna, sardines, and mackerel.

Vegetarian sources of Omega-3 — which must be refrigerated and not heated before consuming — include flax seeds, evening primrose, and borage oil.

- **Omega-6** essential fatty acid is found in mother's milk, organ meats, lean meats, safflower, sunflower, green leafy vegetables, legumes, and Spirulina.

Using antioxidants as anti-aging agents

Oxidation is a natural process that makes objects from food to metal decay. Cut an apple in half, come back a half-hour later, and you'll see that the apple has turned brown. Leave a piece of metal outdoors long enough, and it will rust.

Juicing your way to better nutrition

While surfing television channels in the past, you may have seen an infomercial by Jack La Lanne that touts the benefits of juicing fruits and vegetables to get optimal nutrition from your foods. La Lanne, a pioneer in the field of health and fitness who's now in his 90s, claims that the secret to his longevity is exercise and drinking plenty of fruit and vegetable juice. La Lanne is a dynamic and inspiring example of how important a healthy diet in combination with a well-balanced exercise program really is to longevity and vitality.

Juicing is a great way to include plenty of antioxidants and an array of nutrients in your diet. And it's easy. All you need is high-quality produce and a good juicer. You can buy recipe books for juicing, and your juicer may come with a recipe book to help you get started.

Follow these guidelines to make delicious and nutritious juices in your home:

- Wash all produce before juicing.

- Use only fresh fruits and vegetables, and, whenever you can, buy organic, unsprayed produce.

- Remove pits, seeds, and stems, but use the skins of fruits such as apples and peaches. You may be tempted to peel them, but the skins are full of vitamins and minerals.

- Don't juice bananas and avocados because of their low water content. You can, however, blend them with other fruits and vegetables in juices.

- Use greens, carrots, parsley, bell peppers, celery, and beets to add color to your juices. Color makes the juice more appetizing.

- Use apples, pears, grapes, and melons to sweeten your juice.

- Add a spoonful of juice pulp to your glass before you stir and drink to get more fiber in your diet.

- Make only enough juice for one day, and try to drink it immediately after juicing. Refrigerate juice immediately if you can't drink it right away.

Oxidation also occurs in your body as part of the aging process. When oxygen interacts with your cells, it can cause damage. In most cases, your body replaces the cells, but 1 to 2 percent of the cells are damaged in the course of the replacement process, and these cells produce *free radicals* — unstable, highly reactive molecules with unpaired electrons. Free radicals can injure cells and damage DNA, setting the stage for diseases such as cancer. Antioxidants can help reduce free-radical damage.

Examples of antioxidants include berries, prunes, plums, and raisins. Among vegetables, you can't go wrong with kale, spinach, Swiss chard, broccoli, and Brussels sprouts. Be sure to include antioxidants in your diet. In addition to helping your overall health, antioxidants help your body recover from exercising, especially useful after a yoga-with-weights workout.

Developing Good Eating Habits

Good eating habits are almost as important as good dietary habits for your health and ability to benefit from exercise. In other words, it's not only what you eat, but also how you eat that makes the difference in your health program.

Here are some ideas for developing good eating habits:

✔ **Eat slowly, and savor your food.** Savor each bite, feel its texture, and enjoy its flavor. Chewing releases digestive enzymes in your saliva and helps dissolve the food for digestion. It also permits you to absorb your food better and get the energy you need for yoga-with-weights exercising.

✔ **Eat small portions.** Don't overload your system. Fill half your stomach with food, one quarter with liquid, and then stop. Leave the table a little hungry, but satisfied, rather than stuffed like a big, fat chair. You want to get the nutrients you need for exercising, but you don't want to overdo it.

In the yoga tradition, teachers recommend that you use your hand as a measurement for food. Your palm, held gently like a cup with your fingers together, is considered the right measurement for a food serving. Eating enough to fit in your cupped hand is a nice way to judge the size of a moderate meal. (You can add veggies and salad for a fuller meal.)

✔ **Eat small meals, but eat more often.** Eating small meals throughout the day is easier on your digestive system. By eating this way, you can regulate your energy level at all times of the day, ensuring that you'll always have energy in reserve to start working out.

✔ **Don't be afraid to snack.** You don't need to be embarrassed about feeling hungry when you eat a diet of fresh and whole foods. You can always have something from the whole-foods categories (see "Following Guidelines for Healthy Eating" earlier in this chapter). To keep hunger at bay, snack on fruits and vegetables, small amounts of protein, or whole grains and small amounts of cereal or oatmeal. Taking in enough fluid daily is also helpful so that you don't overeat. You may be thirsty, but your thirst shows up as hunger, so have a glass of water when in doubt and then have something light and healthy if you're still hungry. You should also consider drinking warm tea or vegetable and fruit juice.

Hunger is your body's signal to eat, but most people are unacquainted with this very basic sensation because they may be overeating throughout the day. Appetite is healthy. Tune in to your body's signals, and give it what it needs.

✔ **Make fresh salads and brothy vegetable soups a mainstay in your diet.** These foods are simple to prepare and good to eat, and they give you the energy you need to work out.

Putting your body through detox

Once or twice a year, you should consider undergoing a cleansing and purification diet. Your body is your vehicle for life, so once in a while it pays to clean the machine. Periods of cleansing with natural and water-rich fresh foods clean out old debris in your body at a deep level. Cleansing and purification diets can help you shed unwanted weight and recover your energy and vitality while detoxifying and cleansing your body. In regard to detox diets, Dr. Elson Haas, author of *The New Detox Diet Book: Staying Healthy with Nutrition* (Celestial Arts) and *Vitamins For Dummies* (Wiley), suggests maintaining metabolic balance by maximizing nutrition and eliminating toxins. For a list of books about cleansing and purification diets and for books and Web sites about eating right, see the appendix.

Chapter 14

Addressing Body Aches and Pains

. . . .

In This Chapter

▶ Examining the cause of chronic muscle pain

▶ Relieving pain in your neck and shoulders

▶ Focusing on back pain and discomfort

▶ Loosening tension in your hips

▶ Adding strength and flexibility to your hamstrings and quads

. . . .

Chronic muscle pain interferes with your quality of life. It prevents you from sleeping and taking part in the activities that you like to do. The pain can appear when you least expect it — when you bend over to pick up an envelope you dropped or when you reach for the cereal box in the cupboard. The pain is a handicap that prevents you from enjoying your life. It does nothing less than steal your freedom.

This chapter explains what causes chronic muscle pain and, more importantly, how yoga with weights can help address it. The exercises we provide focus on the parts of the body where most people experience pain and discomfort — the neck, shoulders, hips, lower and upper back, hamstrings, and quadriceps.

We recommend you use the Complete Breath described in Chapter 4 when you perform the exercises in this chapter.

What Causes Chronic Muscle Pain Anyway?

Essentially, your nervous system uses chronic muscle pain to tell you that something in your body isn't right or is out of balance. As if you didn't know already, pain's job is to grab your attention. Muscle pain is a message telling you to change something about your body — the way you stand or sit, what you eat, or how you live your life, for example. Pain tells you to pause, to be more careful, and to be more respectful of your body. Look at it this way: If you touch a hot stove, the pain you feel in your fingertips tells you to move your hand away from the flames. Chronic pain grabs your attention and holds it with a firm, steady grip, but the message that chronic pain sends is harder to interpret. You feel the pain, but you aren't quite sure what's causing it.

Constant, unrelieved muscle pain occurs when you ignore or stop listening to your body signals and continue the behavior that causes the pain. For example, sitting slumped at a computer for hours puts tremendous pressure and strain on your neck and shoulders. You hyperextend your muscles and stretch them out of alignment. Over time, these muscles lose their elasticity and tone and become hardened and rigid. They feel sore, and you experience chronic pain in your neck and shoulders.

Weak muscles that lose their tone and strength can't properly support the skeletal system. Lack of movement and flexibility can also be a factor in reducing elasticity in the connective tissue of your muscles, and this can cause muscle stiffness, rigidity, and pain. For example, many kinds of back pain are caused by weak belly muscles. Your belly muscles are crucial for supporting your back. Without them, you couldn't sit up or stand up straight. If your belly muscles become lax, a chain reaction occurs. The muscles along your spine become lax and nonsupporting as well, which can translate into a sore back.

Yoga with weights is an excellent way to address chronic muscle pain. The slow, relaxed movements help to open up tight and stiff areas of your body. The exercises also strengthen your body so that your musculoskeletal system gets the support it needs from different muscles. In the remainder of this chapter, we show you how to focus on different parts of your body to relieve chronic muscle pain with yoga-with-weights exercises.

Sleeping in spite of neck or back pain

The position in which you sleep can cause neck or back pain or aggravate already painful areas.

If you have neck pain, consider sleeping with a *neck pillow* (sometimes called a *cervical pillow;* the cervical is the top portion of the spine that forms the back of your neck). This pillow supports the curve created by your shoulders, neck, and head. It takes some of the weight from your neck so that your muscles can rest and recuperate.

If you suffer from back pain, take some of the weight off your spine when you sleep. Try lying on your back with a small pillow under your knees. If you prefer sleeping on your side, place a pillow between your knees to relieve your spine of a portion of your body weight. It can take time (for plenty of trial and error), but finding the right mattress is sometimes the cure for back pain. Sleeping on a firm mattress often makes a difference. If you haven't found one, put a half-inch of plywood under your mattress for support.

Diseases such as chronic fatigue syndrome (CFS), Parkinson's disease, and fibromyalgia can also cause chronic muscle pain. Pain can also be a side effect of some prescription drugs. If you're concerned about chronic muscle pain, be sure to consult your doctor.

Managing the Pain in Your Neck

What causes neck pain? Usually, weakness in the muscles of the neck is the culprit, although abnormal sleeping positions, injury, and poor posture can also be causes.

If you have acute pain in your neck, we advise you to consult your healthcare provider for an evaluation and physical-therapy referral.

To relieve neck pain, you can perform the following stretching exercise, which is designed to strengthen your neck muscles. It tones the posterior muscles of your neck, opens up your upper chest, and tones the muscles along your spine. The exercise creates an isolated muscle contraction that helps to maintain the natural curve of your neck and strengthen the supporting muscles around your neck.

Don't attempt this exercise if you've recently had whiplash or compressions in your sternum or vertebrae from an accident of some kind. Consult your healthcare provider for clearance before you attempt strengthening exercises.

Grab your hand weights for this stretching exercise and follow these steps:

1. **Lie on your back with your knees bent, your feet flat on the floor, your elbows bent and at your sides, and the weights in your hands with your palms facing inward.**

   This is the starting position. Engage the muscles of your belly for support.

2. **Press into your elbows and, using the muscles in the backs of your arms, lift your shoulders and back off the ground; lift your chin as well while you arch your back (see Figure 14-1).**

   In this position, the lumbar curve of your lower back lifts up toward your navel, and your belly pulls in and up. Lift your shoulders and chest up, and widen your collarbone. Don't throw yourself into this position; lift your body slowly.

   You should feel the back of your head pressing into the floor and the muscles in the back of your neck engaging.

3. **Hold this pose for three full breaths and then relax back to the starting position (see Step 1).**

   Take slow, relaxed breaths. If you can't hold the pose for three full breaths, hold it as long as you can. (Chapter 4 explains various breathing techniques you can employ.)

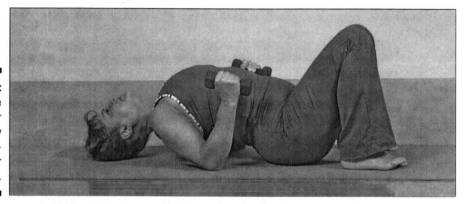

Figure 14-1: Manage the pain in your neck by strengthening your muscles.

Loosening Your Stiff Shoulders

Stiff and sore shoulders are common because so many people carry stress in their shoulders. After all, you "carry all your troubles on your shoulders" and "shoulder your responsibilities." Your shoulders bear plenty of weight — the metaphorical kind and the physical kind — and they can become stiff from lack of movement and chronic tension that builds over time. You probably see people who shrug all the time because they carry so much stress in their shoulders.

Tightness and pain in the shoulders are common because it's so easy to slump your shoulders as you sit at a desk or drive your car, especially if you spend much time at these activities. The average person drives a car or sits in front of a computer for many hours each day.

If you've had a shoulder injury to your rotator cuff or shoulder girdle area, relaxing and loosening the muscles of your shoulders is especially difficult. Because you can't move your shoulders as much as you used to, your shoulders get even stiffer. Over time, you may experience chronic pain because your shoulders have lost their range of motion.

For desk dwellers, truck drivers, and rehabbers alike, the following stretching exercise is designed to relieve discomfort in your shoulders and increase your shoulders' range of motion so your muscles can loosen up.

Grab one hand weight and follow these steps:

1. **Lie on your back with your knees bent and your feet flat on the floor; hold the weight in both hands above your chest with your elbows bent (see Figure 14-2a).**

   This is the starting position. Engage your abdominal muscles for support.

2. **Without turning your head, slowly move the weight to the right side of your body until your right elbow touches the floor (see Figure 14-2b).**

   Feel the backside of your left shoulder — your *trapezius* muscle — loosening and opening up. A nice feeling, no?

   If you also have some discomfort in your neck, you can move your head to the side as you lower the weight and watch the weight as it moves toward the floor. This loosens the muscles on the sides of your neck. You can also loosen your neck muscles by turning your head in the opposite direction.

3. **Take four slow breaths in this position.**

   Inhale to a count of four and exhale to a count of four when you take the breaths. Feel your shoulder muscles loosening. (Chapter 4 presents many yoga breathing techniques you can put into action.)

4. **Move the weight back to the starting position (see Figure 14-2a).**

Pause to rest, and then repeat this exercise by moving the weight to the left side of your body.

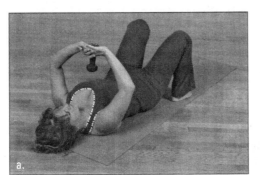

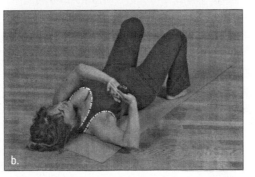

Figure 14-2:
A single hand weight can help you loosen your shoulders.

Relieving Back Discomfort and Pain

You can often blame poor muscle conditioning for back pain. Weak abdominal muscles and weak lower back muscles cause pain that makes it hard to bend down or sit for long periods of time. If weak muscles aren't the problem, musculoskeletal imbalances caused by poor posture can also bring about back pain and back discomfort.

Because back discomfort can have different causes, no single exercise can help relieve the pain all the time. If you experience an acute injury to your back or a recent onset of severe pain, consult your healthcare provider. He or she may be able to give you exercises specific to your injury.

Back pain is an instance when paying attention and listening to your body is essential. Try to find out what's causing your back pain and what you can do — sit in a different way, sleep in a different position, and so on — to alleviate it.

Because no single exercise can alleviate back pain, we offer you three stretching exercises in the pages that follow in the hope that one will do the trick. We present one exercise that addresses back stiffness, one that addresses lower back pain, and one that focuses on your lumbar region. Try out all three and see which works best on your back.

Stretching back stiffness

Your back is a common repository of stress, and stress is a common cause of stiffness. The following stretching exercise is excellent for ironing out stiffness in your back. It increases blood circulation in your back and relieves the stress you carry there.

Grab your hand weights and follow these steps:

1. **Stand with your feet below your hips, your toes pointing forward, and the weights hanging at your sides with your palms facing inward.**

   Engage your belly muscles from the start; you need them to support your spine.

2. **Inhaling to a count of four, slowly roll your shoulders up and forward (see Figure 14-3a).**

   This is the starting position.

3. **Exhaling to a count of four, bend your knees slightly and roll your torso forward, letting the weights hang down in front of you (see Figure 14-3b).**

Your neck, head, and shoulders should be loose and relaxed in this position. Let the weights pull your torso forward and lengthen your spine. Keep your feet parallel to one another, with both feet pointed straight ahead, as you introduce movement into the exercise.

If it feels comfortable, you can remain in this position with the weights hanging down and your torso rolled forward for three or four full breaths (inhaling and exhaling to counts of four). You can really stretch out your spine this way.

4. **Inhaling to a count of four and pressing through your legs, stand up and roll your shoulders up, back, and down as you return to the starting position (see Figure 14-3a).**

   Feel the breath filling your lungs as you return to the upright position.

5. **Exhale to a count of four as you rest in the starting position.**

   Concentrate on the moment as the breath — and your tension — leaves your body.

Do this exercise six to eight times, pause to rest, and then repeat the exercise another six to eight times.

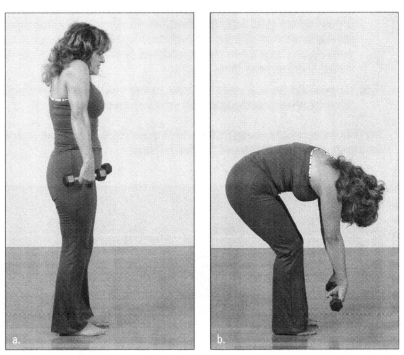

Figure 14-3: This stretching technique relieves tension and pain in your back and spine.

Easing lower back pain

Strong belly muscles help support your lower back and reduce your risk of stiffness and injury. The following stretching exercise is designed to open up your lower back to relive tension and strengthen your belly muscles and the muscles of your inner thighs and back — muscles that support your back, especially the lower part.

You need both ankle weights for this stretching exercise. When you're ready, follow these steps:

1. **Lie on your back with your right knee bent and tucked toward your chest, your fingers interlaced slightly below your knee, and your left leg extended straight out.**

   This is the starting position. Make sure your belly muscles are engaged right away.

2. **As you exhale to a count of four, press your knee into your hands as you raise your head and shoulders off the ground (see Figure 14-4).**

   Keep your left leg flat on the floor. Feel your belly, back, and inner-thigh muscles working.

   If you feel up to it, hold this position for three full breaths (inhale and exhale to counts of four) to really work your belly muscles and stretch your back. If you have knee problems, try holding your leg with your hands behind your knee.

3. **As you inhale to a count of four, lower your head and shoulders to the floor to return to the starting position (see Step 1).**

Do this exercise six to eight times with your right leg, pause to rest, and then do six to eight repetitions with your left leg.

Figure 14-4:
Wring the pain and tension from your lower back by strengthening your core.

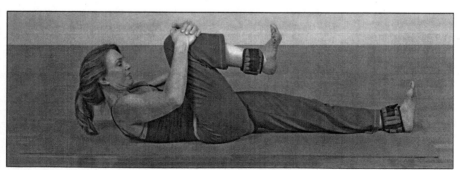

Targeting your lumbar region

Loosely defined, the *lumbar region* is your lower back, an area that often gets sore and emits pain. The region comprises the five lumbar vertebrae between your pelvis and the back of your rib cage. The following stretching exercise is designed to strengthen the muscles that support your lumbar region and loosen your back and spine as a whole to relieve pain.

Strap on your ankle weights for this stretching exercise. When you're ready, follow these steps:

1. **Lie on your back with your knees bent, your feet flat on the floor, and your arms at your sides with your palms flat on the ground (see Figure 14-5a).**

   This is the starting position. Engage your abdominal muscles right away.

2. **Inhaling to a count of four, lift your lower back toward the ceiling as you press into your feet and hands (see Figure 14-5b).**

   Make sure your buttocks, shoulders, and head remain on the floor.

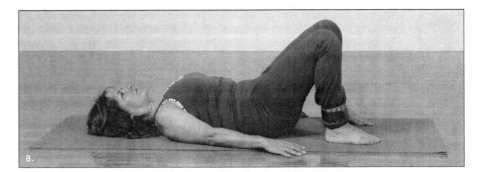

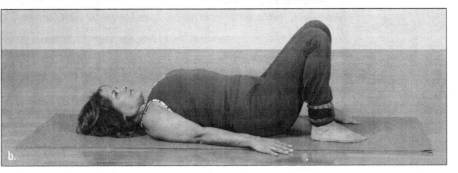

Figure 14-5:
This stretching exercise strengthens your lumbar region.

3. **Exhaling to a count of four, lower your back to the floor to return to the starting position (see Figure 14-5a).**

   Keep your abdominal muscles engaged as you lower your back to the rhythm of your breathing.

Do this exercise six to eight times, pause to rest, and then do six to eight more repetitions.

Alleviating Hip Pain

Any number of injuries can cause hip pain: a pulled groin from an overextension of your legs, tightness in your back, and arthritis, to name a few. Even mild athletic activities can cause hip pain if you forget to stretch before diving in. In the course of a normal day, you don't stretch your hips. When you bend over to pick up some trash, for example, you stretch your hamstrings, but no day-to-day activity stretches your hips. You have to make the extra effort.

Many people experience discomfort when they first start stretching their hips in yoga-with-weights exercises — especially men, who often have tight and rigid hips. As you do hip-stretching exercises, listen carefully to your body, and stretch enough to relieve muscle tension but not so much that you strain your hips.

The following stretching exercise is designed to loosen the muscles of your hips. It isn't easy, but if you stick with it, your hips will start to defrost in no time.

Strap on your ankle weights and follow these steps:

1. **Lie on your back with your right leg bent, your left hand grasping your right knee, and your right hand to your side in the T position.**

   This is the starting position. Your left leg should remain straight as you lie down.

2. **Exhaling to a count of four, roll your right leg over your left leg (see Figure 14-6).**

   Continue to hold your knee with your left hand, and gently press your knee down. Move slowly, and feel your hip muscles stretching and filling with lightness and space as you move your leg.

3. **Inhaling to a count of four, return to the starting position (see Step 1).**

   Instead of returning to the starting position right away, you can try holding your leg in the rollover position for three or four full breaths (inhaling and exhaling to counts of four). You'll find by the third breath that you're really giving your hip a workout.

Do this exercise six to eight times with each leg, pause to rest, and then do six to eight more repetitions with each leg.

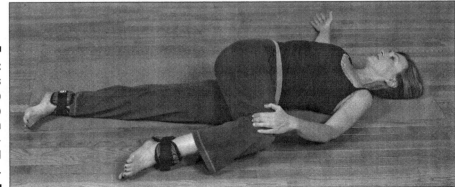

Figure 14-6:
Use this very hip exercise to stretch your oft-neglected hip muscles.

Lengthening Your Hamstrings with a Stretch

The *hamstrings* are the muscle groups that run from your "sitting bones" in the back of your upper legs to slightly below your knees. If you don't have strong or limber hamstrings, you're subject to knee pain, torn cartilage, and poor posture. Tight hips, a tight back, and tight calves can cause your hamstrings to be tight. Over time, chronic tight hamstrings can alter the curvature of your lower back, causing a flattening of your lumbar spine. Tight hamstrings also prevent you from bending over comfortably and touching your toes. In fact, you know your hamstrings are too tight if bending down is uncomfortable for you.

Hamstring tightness in and of itself doesn't cause pain in your hamstrings; most often, tight hamstrings are related to lower back weakness or stiffness. If the muscles of your inner thighs are weak, they don't provide enough support to your pelvic girdle, which puts additional stress on your back and legs, including your hamstrings. In many cases, lower back problems don't resolve themselves until your hamstrings are adequately stretched.

The object of the following stretching exercise is to work your hips and back, and in doing so, loosen and open your hamstrings.

If you have a torn hamstring, do this exercise very carefully. Stretching can help the muscle heal, but overstretching can further damage it. If you feel sharp pain or excessive burning, retreat from the exercise. Only you can tell when your body is ready to push a little farther.

You need ankle weights for this exercise. When you're ready, follow these steps:

1. **Lie on your back with your knees bent, your feet flat on the floor, and your hands at your sides.**

2. **Lift your right knee as close as possible to your chest, and grasp the back of the knee with both hands.**

   This is the starting position.

3. **Straighten your right leg as if you want to press it into the ceiling (see Figure 14-7).**

   Spread your toes wide and press through your foot as you lift your leg. Press your *quad* (the top of your upper leg) to ensure that your hamstring muscle lies closer to the bone where it has optimal lengthening ability.

   Your left leg should be bent if it makes it easier for your right leg to lengthen and stretch. For a better stretch, you can keep your left leg flat on the floor; however, most people are too tight to stretch this way. Having your left leg bent and your left foot on the floor keeps your hips and pelvis stable.

4. **Take three or four deep, full breaths in this position.**

   Feel your hamstring stretching. (Chapter 4 gives you many breathing techniques to choose from.)

5. **Bend your right leg to return to the starting position (see Step 2).**

Repeat this exercise with your left leg. Rest when you need to rest, and stretch as much as you need to in order to feel your hamstrings open up.

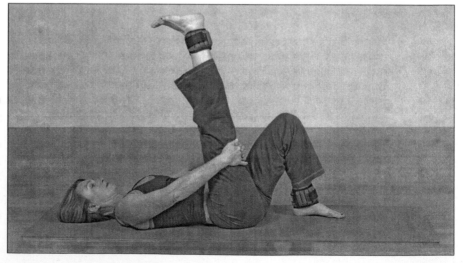

Figure 14-7:
Stretching your hamstrings feels great and is good for the health of your back.

Stretching Out Your Quads

The *quads,* also known as the quadriceps, are the large muscles on the top of your upper legs. They're one of the most important muscle groups because you work your quads when you walk, run, and jump. Strong quads make for strong knee joints, and having loosened quads prevents injury. When your quads are too tight, it puts pressure on your hamstrings, which makes your hamstrings more susceptible to injury. Most people experience pain in their quadriceps because they've lost flexibility in this area. It's important to stretch and warm up your quads before you work out, no matter what kind of exercise you intend to do.

The following two yoga-with-weights exercises strengthen, stretch, and lengthen your quad muscles and give greater stability to your knees.

Standing quad stretcher

Strap on your ankle weights for the following exercise. When you're ready, follow these steps:

1. **Stand behind a chair, holding the top of the chair with your left hand.**

   This is the starting position.

   We highly recommend that you put the chair against a wall, or else it could slide during the exercise, and you may slide to the ground with it. Don't follow the model's lead in Figure 14-8; she's a daredevil.

2. **Bend your right knee and grasp your right foot with your right hand, bringing your heel as close to your buttocks as you comfortably can (see Figure 14-8).**

   For a deeper stretch, use your left hand to hold your right foot. Remember to engage your belly muscles; doing so helps support your back.

3. **Hold this pose for four breaths, and then lower your leg to the starting position (see Step 1).**

   As you inhale and exhale, concentrate on your quad muscles loosening.

Repeat this exercise with your left leg.

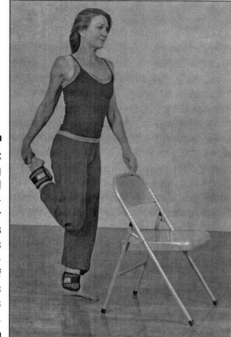

Figure 14-8:
Stretching
and
strengthen-
ing your
quads
improves
the per-
formance of
your legs
from hips
to toes.

Sitting quad stretcher

TIP

For the following quadriceps exercise, you can put a towel or blanket under your feet or between your buttocks and heels if that makes sitting easier.

You need ankle weights for this exercise, but don't strap them on. When you're ready, follow these steps:

1. **Sit on your heels with your knees bent, your feet underneath your buttocks, and the ankle weights resting on your thighs (see Figure 14-9).**

   This is the starting position (and the only position, really). Rest your arms by your sides.

2. **Take three or four slow breaths.**

   The number of breaths you take depends on how comfortable you are in the sitting position. Feel your quads release as you exhale. This exercise not only helps loosen your quads, but also stretches your knee joints.

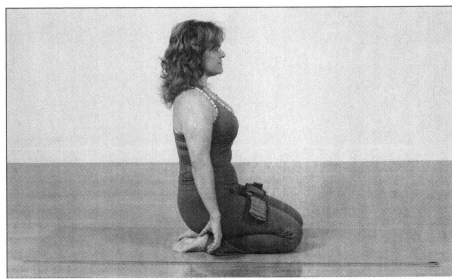

Figure 14-9:
Feel your quads stretching in this meditative pose.

To stretch your quads even more, you can place the ankle weights on your thighs and then gently lean backward, keeping your abdominal muscles engaged to protect your back and legs. You can also try bending forward over your legs for a nice hip and back opener.

Chapter 15

Toning and Focusing on Different Body Areas

....

In This Chapter

▶ Devising your own yoga-with-weights workout

▶ Examining muscle groups and exercises that give them the best workout

....

*T*his chapter explains how yoga with weights can help you strengthen and tone different parts of your body — your legs, arms, shoulders, torso, chest, belly, and buttocks. Sorry, yoga with weights can't exactly strengthen and tone your brain, although it does keep you guessing about what exercise you may come up with next. This chapter is strictly for the body. It's for people who want to target a particular part of their body to tone it, make it look better, or increase its range of motion.

We also give instructions here for creating your own workout. If you spend any time with yoga with weights, you soon discover which exercises work best for you, make you feel stronger, and make you feel better. Suppose you were to gather your favorite exercises into a single workout. To do that, what do you need to know? As we explain in this chapter, you can't do the exercises in just any order, because you have to start slow and finish slow. And you also have to be careful to include the right mix of exercises in the batch. Keep reading if you want to personalize your yoga-with-weights training and take it to another level.

Working out target areas every *other* day is best, because it gives your muscles enough time to recover. Resting your muscles is a bit like sleep. After they're rested, the muscles have more endurance and stamina. You can exercise them harder at the next workout.

Creating Your Own Workout

When you've spent a lot of time doing yoga with weights, when you've done all the workouts and you're well acquainted with the exercises, you may consider creating your own workout. Why not? You know which exercises make you feel healthiest. You know which exercises challenge you the most. If you asked a personal trainer to devise a yoga-with-weights workout especially for you, he or she would charge $50 an hour or more. Creating the workout on your own costs considerably less than that, although it does require a bit of thought on your part. This chapter gives you the tools to create a powerful practice on your own.

Creating your own workout isn't as simple as choosing your favorite exercises and doing them one at a time. As you create a workout that focuses on the parts of the body that matter to you, you have to consider warming up, breathing, the sequence of exercises, the transitions between exercises, meditating, and how often to work out.

In Chapter 16, we present workouts tailor-made for swimming, tennis, baseball, and other popular sports. If your goal is to design a yoga-with-weights workout program so you can play better in the sport you love, turn to Chapter 16.

Warming up

Many people like to jump in and start exercising, but you should always start a workout with warm-up exercises. To begin your custom-made workout, choose some warm-up exercises from Chapter 6. These exercises take only a minute to do, but warm-ups are essential to keep from being injured and to prepare yourself mentally for your workout.

Do one warm-up exercise for each area of your body — your shoulders, back, arms, and legs. If an area of your body is especially stiff or needs attention, do two or three warm-up exercises from Chapter 6 for that area. Besides their physical benefits, the warm-ups help you begin focusing on your yoga-with-weights workout. They put you in the right mindset for exercising.

Breathing

We give instructions for inhaling and exhaling in each exercise we present in this book. Breathing correctly is extremely important in a yoga-with-weights workout. In yoga with weights, you work from the breath into the movement during each exercise. Breathing is so important, in fact, that we select a specific breathing technique for each workout in this book. As part of designing your own workout, choose a breathing technique of your own. Chapter 4 explains the Complete Breath, the Ocean Breath, and other breathing techniques.

When choosing a breathing technique, consider what type of workout you've created for yourself and select the right breath to go with it. For example, if yours is a dynamic workout, choose the Ocean Breath because it will rev your engine. Go with the Complete Breath if your workout is more even-tempered. Try the Cleansing Breath to get your focus and breath control going.

You can tell whether you're working too hard or an exercise is too strenuous by listening to the sound of your breathing. If you can't maintain a steady rhythm as you breathe, or if you start holding your breath, ease back a bit. Work at an easier level until you develop your competence. Holding your breath and breathing unsteadily are signs that you're trying too hard or pushing too far. By focusing on your breathing, you always know when you need to rest and whether you're exercising correctly.

Sequencing

In yoga-with-weights exercising, *sequencing* is the order of exercises in a workout routine. The object is to create a deliberate sequence that ends with you feeling refreshed, alert, and vital. To that end, here are guidelines for developing an exercise sequence for your workout:

1. **Start slowly.**

   Always start with two or three easy exercises. Don't challenge yourself especially hard in the early going. Use your first few exercises as a time to get into the flow of the routine and center yourself. Use a few of the warm-up exercises found in Chapter 6 to prepare yourself first. Then move into a few of the standing exercises to get a sense of breath and flow.

2. **Peak two-thirds of the way through the routine.**

   When you feel energized, move into exercises that offer a challenge and take you into new areas of personal development. Save your hardest exercises — back-bending and abdominal exercises — for two-thirds of the way through. This way, you have ample time to cool down before the meditation period at the end of the workout.

3. **End slowly.**

   Save one or two easy exercises for the end of the routine. Gentle twists, seated exercises, forward bends, and stretches work nicely here. Ideally, you should start with standing exercises and end with sitting exercises, because sitting exercises are easier to do. Ending with a sitting exercise helps you cool down for the meditation at the end of the workout (see the "Ending with meditation" section later for more information).

Try not to work the same muscles in back-to-back exercises. For example, don't do two exercises in a row that work your shoulders. If you give your muscles a rest during a routine, they can work that much harder when you call upon them later on. By the end of the workout, you should feel a nice quality of balance from head to toe.

Transitioning between exercises

What you do between yoga-with-weights exercises is nearly as important as the exercises themselves. The object is to create effortless, flowing, graceful transitions between exercises, with as little excess movement as possible. The entire yoga philosophy is not about abrupt stops and starts, but going seamlessly from one exercise to the next. Done correctly, your workout feels as if it was choreographed, because you pass so gracefully from exercise to exercise. Experiment and tinker with the exercise sequence in your workout until you get it just right. Keep in mind that the breathing serves as the bridge, creating the seamless transitions, and moves you from one action to the next.

By paying attention to transitions as well as exercises, you can carry vitality, strength, and endurance from one exercise to the next. With enough attention to transitions, you can turn your yoga-with-weights workout into a seamless flow with all the postures connected through balance and breath.

In their daily lives, yoga masters attempt to take this smooth transition notion a step further. They try to make all transitions in their lives — transitions from one activity to the next and even from one thought to the next — pass smoothly and gracefully. Yoga is a quality of consciousness, a quality of breath awareness that you can carry with you in your daily life as well as in your yoga-with-weights workouts.

Ending with meditation

The meditation at the end of the workout is like a ribbon that ties everything together. In our yoga classes, one or two students always skip out before the meditation period at the end of the workout. If it weren't for the fact that the meditation is meant to be quiet and contemplative, we would shout at these students: "Hey, wait a minute! Yes, I'm talking to you! You're missing one of the best parts of the class — perhaps even the most important one, the one you may need the most!"

Meditation is an excellent opportunity to sit with yourself and your thoughts. It's your chance to take an inner inventory, so to speak, and look within yourself for direction in your life. Meditation requires training and patience, but the rewards are plentiful. It leaves you stronger and wiser. And think about it: If you can't stand to be with yourself in meditation, why should anyone else want to be with you?

Be sure to include a meditation at the end of your workout. A meditation takes only a few moments, integrating all the practices of your workout, as it quiets your body and mind, leaving you feeling refreshed and ready for the rest of your day. With practice, meditation gives you more balance and clarity in your life. Chapter 6 explains what yoga meditation is and gives many different ways and techniques to help you meditate.

Choosing how and when to work out

As tempted as you may be to focus exclusively on one part of your body in your custom-made workout, try to work several parts. Overtraining one part of your body or one muscle group can cause strains and even injuries.

Choose a different workout for each day or every other day of the week, and take a break from exercising on the fourth day. This way, you don't overdo it in the beginning. Instead of a yoga-with-weights workout on your day of rest, go for a walk and do warm-up exercises (see Chapter 6). You need some physical activity every day to stay in good health.

Change your exercise program every three to six weeks. You favor certain muscles — and perhaps overdevelop them — by doing the same exercises all the time. And you can get into an exercise rut and suffer from boredom if you stay with the same routine. By continually adapting your exercise program, you make sure all the areas of your body get enough exercise and continually challenge yourself at yoga with weights.

Targeting Parts of Your Body

Do you want to strengthen your shoulders? Take a couple of inches from your waist? Maybe you want to make your back stronger to help prevent backaches. The remainder of this chapter presents exercises that target different parts of your body — your shoulders, chest, arms, back, belly, hips, buttocks, and legs. Use these yoga-with-weights exercises to put together a workout tailored just for you.

Figures 15-1 and 15-2 show the muscles of the body that we focus on in the following sections.

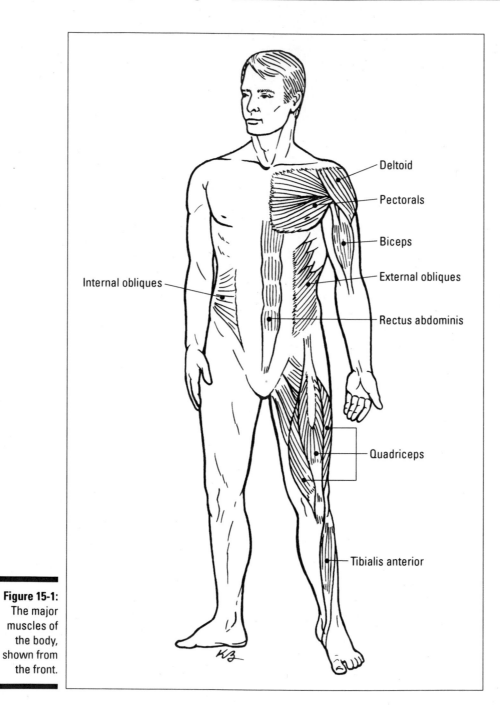

Figure 15-1:
The major
muscles of
the body,
shown from
the front.

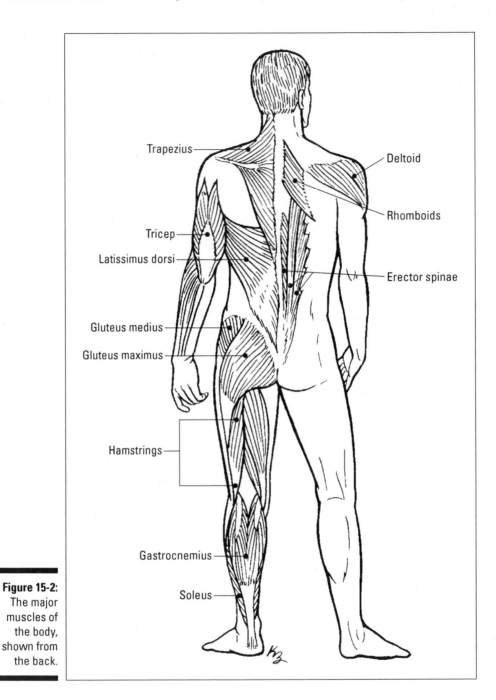

Trapezius

Deltoid

Rhomboids

Tricep

Latissimus dorsi

Erector spinae

Gluteus medius

Gluteus maximus

Hamstrings

Gastrocnemius

Soleus

Figure 15-2:
The major
muscles of
the body,
shown from
the back.

Developing your shoulders

In case you didn't know already, your shoulders are located in the upper torso area where your arms connect to your upper back and chest. Without strong shoulder muscles, you can't have a strong upper body or strong arms. Almost all exercises and activities that work your chest and back also work your shoulders. The shoulders are made up primarily of the deltoid and rotator cuff (refer to Figure 15-3):

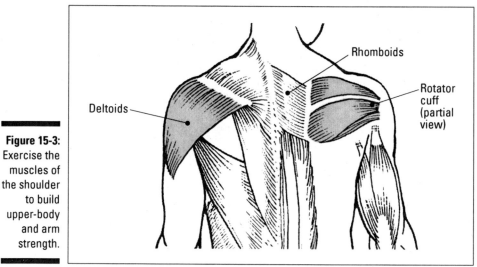

Figure 15-3: Exercise the muscles of the shoulder to build upper-body and arm strength.

© IUSM Office of Visual Media

 ✔ **Deltoid:** This muscle wraps completely around the tops of your arms. It's responsible for rotating the shoulders, rolling the shoulders, and moving the arm in all directions. Strengthening the deltoid can help prevent injuries to the shoulder.

 ✔ **Rotator cuff:** This muscle, which is positioned around your shoulder joint, holds your arm in its socket and keeps the shoulder joint stable when you move your arm. You use this muscle every time you throw a ball or any other object. The rotator cuff is actually the name for four small muscles that work in consort: the subscapularis, teres minor, infraspinatus, and supraspinatus.

Table 15-1 describes exercises from this book that strengthen the muscles of the shoulder or make these muscles more flexible.

Table 15-1		Exercises for Your Shoulders
Chapter	*Exercise*	*What This Exercise Does*
7	Dog	Strengthens your rhomboids below your shoulders that are responsible for holding and supporting your shoulders.
8	Dog to Plank	Strengthens your arms, shoulders, and back of your body, as well as the core muscles of your trunk and torso.
8	Twisted Triangle	Strengthens and conditions your deltoids, rotator cuff, and muscles of your back.
8	Eye of the Needle	Conditions your shoulder girdle and upper back; makes your shoulder and back more flexible.
11	Side Bow	Works your deltoid and shoulder girdle.

Working on your chest

If you look down, you can see your chest. It's the thing that you spill seeds on when you're eating watermelon. The primary muscles of the chest are the pectorals, known affectionately to weightlifters as the "pecs" (see Figure 15-4). These muscles are used for pushing and for squeezing. For example, when you push open a heavy door or hug a tree, you use your pectoral muscles. The pectoralis major flexes, adducts, and rotates your arms medially. When you climb a tree, these muscles draw your body upward. The pectoralis minor draws the scapula, or shoulder blade, downward. For example, when you push yourself up from a chair with your hands and arms, you flex your pectoralis minor. All these muscles work together to create coordinated movement.

Conditioning the pectorals helps lift the chest up. In women, strong pectoral muscles help support the breasts and make them firmer. Table 15-2 lists exercises in this book that you can use to strengthen your pectoral muscles.

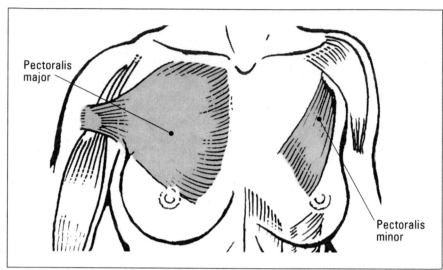

Figure 15-4:
Work on your pectoral muscles to make pushing heavy objects easier.

Table 15-2		Exercises for Your Chest
Chapter	*Exercise*	*What This Exercise Does*
8	Twisted Triangle	Strengthens, conditions, and stretches your chest, back, and arms.
8	Eye of the Needle	Conditions your shoulder girdle and upper back; makes your shoulders and back more flexible.
8	Rise and Shine	Strengthens and conditions your chest, shoulders, back, and arms; lengthens and tones your trunk muscles.
9	Sphinx	Stretches your pectorals by opening up the front of your body and widening your collarbones.
10	Dolphin	Activates your pectorals as you lift from your armpits.
11	Side Bow	Strengthens and stretches your pectorals, back, shoulders, and arms.
11	Press	Strengthens and conditions your chest, arms, shoulders, and upper back.
11	Straddle	Conditions your chest because your arms are extended.

Toning and strengthening your arms

Poor Venus de Milo didn't have any arms, and her yoga-with-weights work-outs focused exclusively on her legs and torso. You, however, are invited to tone and strengthen your arms with yoga-with-weights exercises. As shown in Figure 15-5, the primary muscles of the arm are the biceps and triceps:

- ✔ **Biceps:** These two muscles are found in the front of the upper arm. They are responsible for bending your elbow. Strong biceps are necessary for lifting heavy loads and growing toddlers.

- ✔ **Triceps:** These muscles in back of the upper arm straighten the elbow. You also engage these muscles along with the pectorals when you push with your hands. And you use your triceps when you carry a briefcase, bowling ball, or other heavy object at the end of your extended arm.

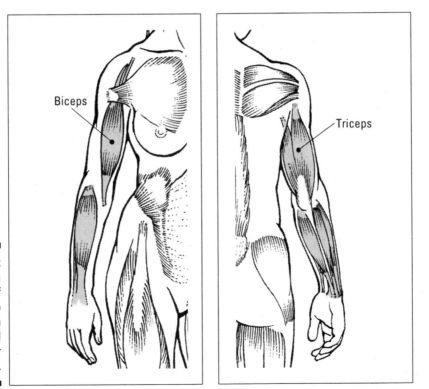

Biceps

Triceps

Figure 15-5:
You use the muscles of your arms to straighten your tie and lift your briefcase.

© IUSM Office of Visual Media

The exercises listed in Table 15-3 help condition the muscles of the arms and wrists.

Table 15-3		Exercises for Your Arms and Wrists
Chapter	*Exercise*	*What This Exercise Does*
7	Exalted Warrior	Works your back, shoulders, biceps, and triceps.
7	Warrior II	Exercises your biceps.
7	Triangle	Works your shoulders, back, and arms.
7	Dog	Offers excellent conditioning and stretching for your arms, wrists, shoulders, back, and legs.
8	Warrior I	Exercises your biceps.
8	Dog to Plank	Conditions and strengthens your entire torso.
9	Child's Pose	Exercises your triceps; stretches out your back and quadriceps in your legs.
10	Swimmer	Strengthens your upper and lower back, shoulders, arms, and chest.
11	Tree	Exercises your triceps and improves your shoulder girdle's range of motion.
12	Staff	Works your arms, chest, abdominals, and back.

Focusing on the back of the torso and spine

Along with your spine, the muscles of your back provide strength and stability for your entire body. For that reason, unless your back is strong, you can't have strong arms or legs, in much the same way that a tree's branches can't grow big unless the trunk is strong enough to support the branches. The muscles on your back are oriented to the vertebrae in your spine. These muscles are consistently shifting, flexing, and relaxing so you can balance. As shown in Figure 15-6, these are the primary muscles of the back of the torso and spine.

✔ **Trapezius:** This muscle is found on each side of your spine. It runs from the neck, across the back of the shoulders, to the middle of your back. You flex it when you lift your shoulders or lift your arm to your side. The trapezius carries stress and for that reason is prone to being tight.

✔ **Rhomboids:** These muscles, also found on each side of the spine, are located in the center of your back. You use them to pull your shoulder blades together and assist in drawing your shoulders down. Strong rhomboids are necessary for good posture and for keeping your back erect.

✔ **Latissimus dorsi:** Known as the "lats" to weightlifters, these large muscles run the length of your back, from below your shoulders to your lower back. You use them to pull yourself over high brick walls and hold boulders over your head. They're also important for good posture, because they keep you from slouching or having rounded shoulders.

✔ **Erector spinae:** These muscles run the entire length of your back. Along with your abdominals, they are responsible for straightening your spine. Back pain is sometimes caused by weak erector spinae and abdominal muscles.

Table 15-4 lists exercises in this book that work the back of your torso and the muscles connected to your spine.

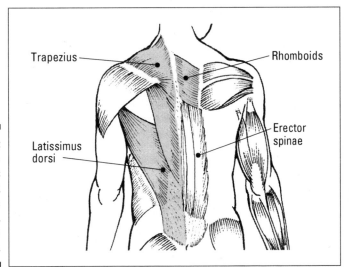

Figure 15-6:
Focus on the muscles of the back to increase strength, stability, and support.

Trapezius

Rhomboids

Erector spinae

Latissimus dorsi

© IUSM Office of Visual Media

Table 15-4		Exercises for the Back of Your Torso
Chapter	*Exercise*	*What This Exercise Does*
7	Dog	Conditions and stretches your arms, wrists, shoulders, upper and lower back, and legs.
7	Airplane	Conditions and strengthens your upper and lower back, shoulders, arms, and abdominals.
7	Cat	Stretches and conditions your back, abdominals, shoulders, arms, and legs.
7	Table	Tones and conditions the muscles of your trunk.
9	Twister	Stretches and tones your back, abdominals, and waistline.
10	Swimmer	Strengthens the core muscles of your trunk and torso.
10	Lift	Offers total-body strengthening and conditioning.
11	Horse	Strengthens your back, abdominals, and the core muscles of your trunk.
11	Dancer	Develops balance and coordination.
12	Cow to Cat	Stretches and tones your back and abdominal muscles.
12	Flying Locust	Strengthens your back, abdominals, arms, and legs.
12	Locust	Strengthens your upper and lower back, and your abdominals.
12	Staff	Strengthens and conditions your upper body, back, spine, and abdominals.
12	Pearl	Strengthens and tones your back and abdominal muscles.
12	Belly Crunch	Strengthens your back and abdominal muscles.

Engaging your belly muscles

Most people exercise their belly muscles — better known as the abdominal muscles — because they want a flatter stomach and a trimmer figure. However, these muscles serve purposes besides keeping you trim. Most importantly, they support your spine and back. They also improve your posture (if they're strong). As shown in Figure 15-7, these are the muscles of the belly.

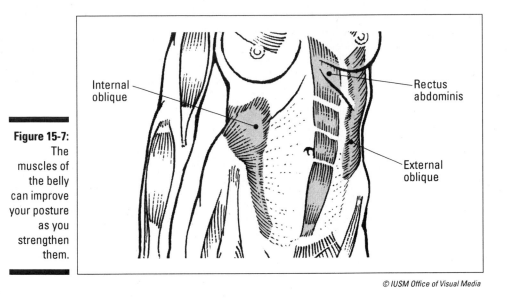

Figure 15-7: The muscles of the belly can improve your posture as you strengthen them.

© IUSM Office of Visual Media

✔ **Rectus abdominus:** This flat sheet of muscle runs from under the chest down to below the navel. You flex this muscle when you bend at the waist or do a sit-up.

✔ **Internal and external obliques:** These muscles run diagonally down the sides of your body and connect to the rectus abdominus. You use them to twist or bend from side to side. Having strong obliques helps support the spine and prevent lower back pain.

We devote an entire chapter of this book to strengthening the belly muscles — Chapter 12. Besides the exercises described there, you can do these exercises to strengthen your belly muscles: the Plow (in Chapter 9) and the Horse (in Chapter 11).

Toning your buttocks and hips

Strengthening the buttocks and hips can help prevent hip and lower back injuries. Our students often ask us for specialized exercises that focus on making their hips more flexible. Because the hips come into play when you walk, sit, and stand, having flexible hips is essential for longevity and for quality of movement throughout your life. As shown in Figure 15-8, these muscles make up the buttocks and hips.

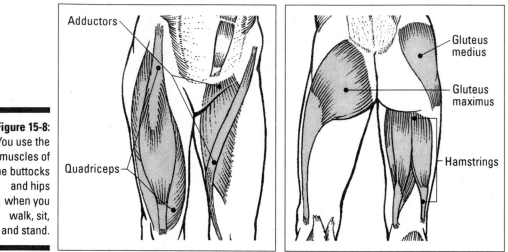

Adductors

Quadriceps

Gluteus medius

Gluteus maximus

Hamstrings

Figure 15-8:
You use the muscles of the buttocks and hips when you walk, sit, and stand.

© IUSM Office of Visual Media

✔ **Gluteus maximus and gluteus medius:** Known as "glutes" to weightlifters, these muscles span the entire width of the buttocks, from the cheek to the derriere (pardon our French). When you jump, climb stairs, or rise out of a chair, you exercise your glutes.

✔ **Hip abductors:** This muscle group is found in the upper quadrant of the hip and buttocks area. You use it when you rotate your hips or move your legs to the side. Weak hip abductors cause you to shuffle when you walk.

✔ **Leg adductors:** These muscles run from the inside of the hip to various points along the inner thigh. You flex these muscles when you move from side to side.

We also should mention the pelvic girdle, which is the boney structure, composed of several fused bones, that surrounds the pelvis. It receives the weight of the upper body and passes it to the lower limbs; it absorbs stress from the lower limbs as well. Keeping the muscles surrounding the pelvic girdle toned and conditioned is necessary for healthy movement and overall stability.

To keep your hips from freezing up and your buttocks from sagging, try out the exercises listed in Table 15-5.

Table 15-5		Exercises for Your Buttocks and Hips
Chapter	*Exercise*	*What This Exercise Does*
7	Cat	Stretches and conditions your back, gluteus muscles, your abdominals, shoulders, arms, and legs; makes your hips more flexible.
7	Bridge	Strengthens, conditions, and stretches your trunk, arms, legs, and gluteus muscles.
7	Table	Strengthens, tones, and conditions your trunk, legs, and gluteus muscles.
7	Frog	Stretches and conditions your inner and outer thigh, your hips, and your pelvic girdle.
8	Runner	Stretches and conditions your hip flexors, legs, back, spine, gluteus muscles, shoulders, and arms.
8	Skater	Strengthens your inner and outer thigh, legs, gluteus muscles, and abdominal muscles.
8	Chair	Offers flexibility and conditioning for your hip flexors, inner and outer thighs, calves, and legs.
9	Plow	Stretches and conditions your hip flexors, abdominals, back, and gluteus muscles.
9	Pigeon	Stretches and conditions your hip flexors, buttocks, and pelvic girdle.
10	Lift	Conditions and strengthens your upper and lower torso, gluteus muscles, and legs.
10	Lightning Bolt	Conditions and tones your back, abdominals, gluteus muscles, and legs.
10	Half Moon	Strengthens your core muscles, gluteus muscles, arms, and legs; develops balance, stability, and coordination.
11	Horse	Strengthens your back, abdominals, and gluteus muscles.
11	Side Bow	Strengthens your core muscles, gluteus muscles, arms, and legs; develops balance, stability, and coordination.
12	Cow to Cat	Stretches and tones your back, gluteus muscles, and abdominal muscles.

Strengthening your legs

Unless you have strong legs, you can't run away from your creditors (just kidding!). Besides enjoying a good walk, the best reason to have strong legs is to prevent common injuries to the knees and ankles. Strong legs are also necessary for balancing. These are the primary muscles of the legs:

- ✔ **Quadriceps:** This is the name for the four muscles on the top of the leg above the knee (refer to Figure 15-1). These muscles are responsible for straightening your leg. They play an important role in walking and running.

- ✔ **Hamstrings:** This group includes three muscles on the back of the upper leg. These muscles bend your knee (refer to Figure 15-2). Working in opposition to your quadriceps, they enable you to walk and run. The hamstrings are especially prone to injury, so you should warm them up before exercising.

- ✔ **Gastrocnemius and soleus:** These muscles, better known as your calves, make up the large, diamond-shaped muscle group on the back of your lower leg (refer to Figure 15-9). You flex this muscle group to stand on your toes and to spring when you jump. The Achilles tendon is connected to this muscle group.

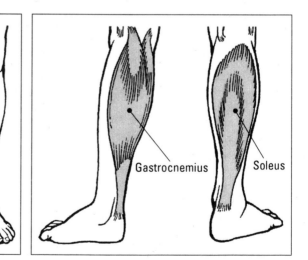

Figure 15-9: Strengthening your leg muscles is an important part of yoga with weights.

Tibialis anterior

Gastrocnemius

Soleus

© IUSM Office of Visual Media

- ✔ **Tibialis anterior:** This muscle runs from the front of your ankle to just below your kneecap (refer to Figure 15-9). You use it to bend your ankle and draw your toes upward. You can get shin splints if this muscle isn't properly conditioned.

- ✔ **Adductor:** This muscle is located in the inner thigh (refer to Figure 15-8). It keeps the hip and pelvis stable and flexes when you move your leg forward.

The exercises listed in Table 15-6 help you strengthen the muscles of your legs.

Table 15-6		Exercises for Your Legs
Chapter	*Exercise*	*What This Exercise Does*
7	Frog	Stretches and conditions your inner and outer thigh, hips, and pelvic girdle.
7	Bridge	Strengthens, conditions, and stretches your trunk, arms, legs, and gluteus muscles.
7	Camel	Tones, conditions, and stretches your legs, buttocks, and abdominal muscles.
7	Exalted Warrior	Strengthens and conditions your entire leg as well as your gluteus muscles, hip flexors, back, and abdominal muscles.
8	Warrior I	Strengthens and conditions your entire leg, gluteus muscles, hip flexors, back, and abdominal muscles.
8	Skater	Strengthens and conditions your entire leg, gluteus muscles, hip flexors, back, abdominals, and your inner and outer thigh.
8	Crow	Strengthens and conditions your entire leg, gluteus muscles, hip flexors, back, and abdominal muscles; stretches your inner and outer thigh.
8	Runner	Stretches and conditions your hip flexors, legs, back, spine, gluteus muscles, shoulders, and arms.
10	Half Moon	Develops balance. stability, and coordination; strengthens your core muscles, gluteus muscles, arms, and legs.
10	Crescent Moon	Develops balance, stability, and coordination; strengthens your core muscles, gluteus muscles, arms, legs, and hip flexors.
11	Eagle	Develops balance, stability, and coordination; strengthens your core muscles, gluteus muscles, arms, legs, and hip flexors.
11	Road Runner	Stretches and conditions your hip flexors, legs, back, spine, gluteus muscles, shoulders, and arms.

Part IV
Personalizing Your Program

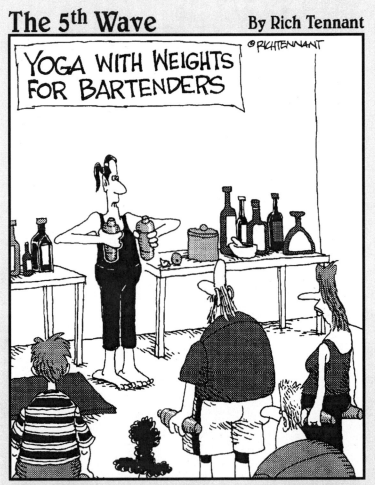

The 5th Wave   By Rich Tennant

YOGA WITH WEIGHTS FOR BARTENDERS

"For this one, you want your cocktail shakers completely filled. I like to use a Mai Tai but you could also use a Zombie or a Purple Hooter."

In this part . . .

One of the great things about exercise and leading a healthy lifestyle is that it's all about you. You can personalize your lifestyle to fit your needs. Part IV is for people who want to make the yoga-with-weights exercise program their own. You can take the workouts from the previous parts of this book and fashion a workout tailored just for you.

We start with some dietary advice. Like all dynamic forms of exercise, yoga-with-weights workouts are more beneficial when you're on a healthy diet. Everyday life places demands on your body, and to meet those demands, you need the right fuel. When you're finished eating, we show you how to address aches and pains in different parts of your body with different yoga-with-weights exercises. We also show you how to tone and strengthen different parts of your body with yoga with weights.

Chapter 16

Improving Your Game

In This Chapter

▶ Addressing stamina and focus for endurance sports

▶ Conditioning your body for team sports

▶ Expanding your range of motion and concentration for ball sports

▶ Giving yourself an edge when it's you against your body

*Y*oga with weights is an excellent training foundation for athletes, no matter which sport you play or how often you participate. Trainers agree that you should *be* in shape for the sport of your choice, not *get* in shape for it. In other words, to have more fun, get more out of a sport, and prevent yourself from being injured, you should be in shape before you begin; you shouldn't use the sport as a means of getting in shape. Yoga with weights can help you get in shape mentally and physically for the sport you love. The weight-bearing exercises, the stretching, the exercises that build stamina, and the exercises that help you develop coordination and balance are ideal for athletes.

Yoga with weights improves your strength, extends your body's range of motion, and releases tension from your muscles. It also trains you to concentrate and focus. You reap the benefits of being completely on the ball and completely in the moment. Most athletes know the moment when time stands still — no thought, no separation, just an expanded sense of being alive, of being whole. Yoga with weights can help you find the zone and play in it more often. Aside from the exercises themselves, the breathing techniques we present give you more control and poise so you can maintain your inner steadiness. You gain self-knowledge, self-study, and self-observation skills that make you a skilled, more balanced athlete.

For each sport we include in this chapter, we provide a yoga-with-weights workout: a series of exercises culled from the different workouts in this book, as well as warm-up exercises from Chapter 6. You don't have to do all the yoga-with-weights exercises or warm-up exercises that we recommend; these exercises are just guidelines. You can choose and create any combination of exercises that feels right to you. All we ask is that you limit the yoga-with-weights exercises to no more than ten at a time. Experiment with all the exercises and select the ones that give you the most satisfaction. Over time, you'll be able to create a workout that suites you and improves your performance in your sport of choice.

Swimming

Swimming is a wonderful activity for toning your upper body, torso, and legs. Unlike cardiovascular activities such as jogging and weight training, swimming doesn't put any stress on your joints because, in effect, you're weightless when you're in the water. Another plus is that the water pressure on your arms and legs benefits your circulatory system.

The yoga-with-weights exercises in Table 16-1 tone and condition the core muscles of your belly and torso and stretch and tone the supporting structures of your shoulders so you can get a longer, smoother, cleaner stroke. You'll also notice better balance and coordination in your kicking legs and more power in your kick.

As you do the exercises, take Complete Breaths (Chapter 4 presents many different breathing techniques). This rhythmic technique will help you be aware of your breathing and get you ready for the rigors of swimming.

Warm-up exercises (see Chapter 6): Back Shoulder Roll, Forward Shoulder Roll, All-Out Hamstring Stretcher, Quad Stretcher, The Big Stretcher, Big Shoulder Release

Table 16-1		A Swimmer's Workout
Chapter	*Exercise*	*Notes*
7	The Camel	Opens up your chest; strengthens your shoulders, arms, and legs; brings flexibility to your shoulders
8	The Eye of the Needle	Brings flexibility to your shoulders and back
8	The Runner	Stretches and tones your back, legs, and arms
9	The Twister	Strengthens and tones your back and abdominal muscles
9	The Child's Pose	Stretches your back, pelvic girdle, quads, and inner thighs; tones and conditions your triceps and shoulder girdle
10	The Lightning Bolt	Gives you strength and a powerful kick
10	The Crescent Moon	Conditions your legs, back, and arms; helps with core strengthening
10	The Swimmer	Strengthens and tones your arms, back, buttocks, legs, and abdomen

Chapter	Exercise	Notes
10	The Lift	Strengthens your arms, back, abdomen, buttocks, and legs
11	The Horse	Strengthens and tones your abdomen, arms, back, buttocks, and legs
11	The Dancer	Helps stretch your quads and the head of your shoulder girdle
11	The Straddle	Opens your pelvic girdle; conditions your back and abdomen; strengthens your biceps
12	The Locust	Strengthens your shoulders, chest, arms, legs, buttocks, and abdominal muscles
12	The Pearl	Works your abdominal muscles and stretches out your spine
12	The Flying Locust	Strengthens and tones the front and back of your body; strengthens your shoulders, arms, chest, legs and buttocks

Running

Running is one of the best cardiovascular workouts you can perform. It increases your lungs' ability to take in oxygen and strengthens your heart. It also helps lower your blood pressure because it maintains the elasticity of your arteries and enables blood to flow more easily through your body; in turn, running increases your stamina, burns calories so you can lose weight, and prevents the bone and muscle loss that accompany aging. Figure 16-1 shows a couple of Sherri's yoga students, Paula Glodowski and Andy Valla, completing an iron-man triathlon.

You can use the yoga-with-weights exercises in Table 16-2 to develop core strength in your abdominal muscles to improve your running performance. These exercises also help you rehabilitate injuries, improve your overall fitness, recover between runs, and rejuvenate your mind and body. Because runners often experience pulled muscles and other injuries in their calves, hamstrings, and groin, we include exercises that condition, stretch, and support those areas. By addressing all these areas through yoga-with-weights exercises, you can prolong your running career.

Warm-up exercises (see Chapter 6): Forward Shoulder Roll, Backward Shoulder Roll, Quad Stretcher, All-Out Hamstring Stretcher

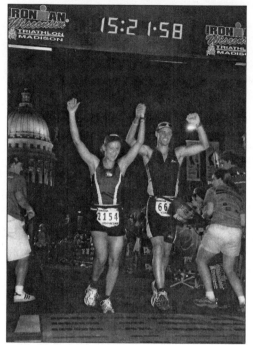

Figure 16-1: Paula Glodowski and Andy Valla, two of Sherri's yoga students, crossing the finish line.

Table 16-2		A Runner's Workout
Chapter	**Exercise**	**Notes**
7	The Rag Doll	Stretches out your legs, back, head, neck, shoulders, and arms
7	The Warrior II	Strengthens your legs, buttocks, trunk, and upper torso
7	The Dog	Offers total-body strengthening and conditioning
7	The Frog	Opens up your groin, hips, and pelvis; stretches and strengthens your legs
8	The Skater	Strengthens and tones your legs, buttocks, abdomen, back, shoulders, and arms; enhances balance and stability
8	The Runner	Strengthens and tones your legs, buttocks, back, shoulders, and arms; enhances balance and coordination

Chapter	Exercise	Notes
8	The Warrior I	Strengthens and tones your legs, buttocks, back, shoulders, and arms; opens up your hips and groin
8	The Rise and Shine	Strengthens and stretches your legs, back, shoulders, and arms; enhances fluidity of movement
9	The Twister	Strengthens and tones your abdomen, sides, and back; opens up your upper chest; stretches your arms
9	The Pigeon	Stretches your hips and groin
9	The Plow	Tones and strengthens your core muscles, legs, and back
10	The Swimmer	Strengthens and tones your arms, back, buttocks, legs, and abdomen
10	The Lightning Bolt	Stretches and tones your arms, back, sides, and legs; enhances balance and stability
11	The Straddle	Stretches your groin, hips, and legs; strengthens your abdomen, back, and biceps
11	The Road Runner	Stretches and strengthens your hamstrings, back, and arms; tones your abdomen; enhances coordination
11	The Dancer	Stretches and tones your legs, quadriceps, and back; conditions your shoulder girdle, arms, and abdomen; develops balance and stability
12	The Cow to Cat	Opens up your back and spine; strengthens and tones your abdomen, legs, buttocks, and core
12	The Love Handler	Stretches your pelvic girdle and legs; tones and conditions your abdomen and sides
12	The Burning Boat	Strengthens and conditions your abdomen, arms, legs, and back
12	The Archer	Strengthens your core; stretches and tones your back and legs

Cycling

Cycling has most of the benefits of running, but you get to cover more ground and see more terrain. It builds your stamina and helps lower your blood pressure. It helps you lose weight, prevents muscle and bone loss, and increases your lungs' capacity to breathe in oxygen. Compared to running, cycling presents fewer risks of injury (unless you're mountain biking or speed racing). And cycling has another benefit apart from exercise — it's a great way to get around without polluting the air you breathe.

In the 1960s, German bike racer Rudi Altig, the "Manheim Colossus," announced to the world that he was a yoga enthusiast. He did yoga exercises before and after races to relax his muscular body and center his mind. Altig was one of the first athletes to embrace yoga as a way to improve his performance in sport.

The exercises in Table 16-3 would make Altig proud. They build strength and condition your whole body, and they give your legs greater range of movement so you can pedal faster and more efficiently. The exercises also strengthen your back, spine, and shoulders so they can support your upper torso as you ride your bike. And because bikers often experience tight hamstrings because of the extra muscle packed into their thighs, these exercises stretch and strengthen your legs. Along with the breathing techniques you see associated with these exercises, the yoga-with-weights alignment principals will help prepare you for the ride of your life.

Warm-up exercises (see Chapter 6): Chin-Chest Tuck, Head Turner, Lateral Neck Release, Backward Shoulder Roll, Forward Shoulder Roll, Side Bender, Wrist Rotator, Hip Twister, Quad Stretcher, All-Out Hamstring Stretcher

Table 16-3		A Cyclist's Workout
Chapter	*Exercise*	*Notes*
7	The Airplane	Strengthens and conditions your legs, back, and arms; enhances balance and stability
7	The Exalted Warrior	Strengthens and conditions your legs, buttocks, back, shoulders, and arms; enhances balance and stability
7	The Dog	Offers total-body strengthening and conditioning
7	The Frog	Stretches your groin, hips, and pelvic girdle; strengthens your legs
8	The Eye of the Needle	Offers flexibility for your shoulders and back

Chapter	Exercise	Notes
8	The Dog to Plank	Strengthens and conditions your whole body, especially your core
8	The Twisted Triangle	Stretches and strengthens your legs, hips, pelvis, back, and sides; tones and conditions your abdomen and arms; develops balance and coordination
9	The Twister	Strengthens and tones your abdomen, sides, and back; opens up your upper torso and chest
9	The Sphinx	Strengthens and tones your upper back, shoulders, and arms; gently stretches your quads; conditions your buttocks
10	The Swimmer	Strengthens and tones your arms, back, buttocks, legs, and abdomen
10	The Dolphin	Strengthens and conditions your upper torso, arms, abdomen, back, and legs; stretches your back and legs
10	The Lift	Strengthens your arms, back, abdomen, buttocks, and legs
11	The Dancer	Helps stretch your quads, back, and shoulder girdle; enhances balance and stability
11	The Road Runner	Strengthens and conditions your hamstrings, legs, abdomen, back, and arms; enhances endurance and coordination
11	The Horse	Offers overall body strengthening and conditioning
11	The Straddle	Stretches your groin, hips, and legs; strengthens your abdomen, back, and biceps
12	The Cow to Cat	Stretches and tones your back and spine; conditions your abdomen, legs, and buttocks
12	The Flying Locust	Strengthens and tones the front and back of your body; strengthens your shoulders, arms, chest, legs, and buttocks
12	The Staff	Strengthens and conditions your abdomen, back, spine, shoulders, hamstrings, and quads
12	The Burning Boat	Offers core abdominal strengthening; builds endurance and stamina

Basketball

Depending on whom you're playing with or against, basketball can be a very grueling exercise. No sport has as much variety of movement as basketball. You run, jump, move sideways, move backward, and occasionally dive to the floor for a loose ball. On account of the variety of movement, basketball works a variety of muscles. It requires excellent stamina and hand-eye coordination, and you have to be physically and mentally quick. The sport is a wonderful cardiovascular activity and a total-body workout.

Whether you play basketball competitively or play for fun, the yoga-with-weights exercises in Table 16-4 help you jump higher for more rebounds and scoring and build your endurance and stamina. "There is no way I could have played as long as I did without yoga," NBA all-time leading scorer Kareem Abdul-Jabbar told *Men's Health* magazine. "My friends and teammates think I made a deal with the devil. But it was yoga that made my training complete."

Warm-up exercises (see Chapter 6): Head Turner, Lateral Neck Release, Backward Shoulder Roll, Forward Shoulder Roll, Side Bender, The Big Stretcher, Wrist Rotator, Hip Twister, Quad Stretcher, All-Out Hamstring Stretcher

Table 16-4		A Baller's Workout
Chapter	**Exercise**	**Notes**
7	Heaven and Earth	Stretches and lengthens your back, sides, arms, and legs
7	The Rag Doll	Releases tension in your head, neck, shoulders, and back; conditions your abdominal muscles, back, and legs
7	The Airplane	Strengthens and conditions your legs, back, and arms; enhances balance and stability
7	The Triangle	Strengthens, stretches, and conditions your legs, hips, back, abdominal muscles, shoulders, and arms
7	The Warrior II	Strengthens and conditions your legs, the core muscles of your trunk and torso, and your shoulders
7	The Dog	Offers total-body strengthening and conditioning
7	The Frog	Stretches your groin, hips, and pelvic girdle; stretches and strengthens your legs

Chapter	Exercise	Notes
8	The Chair	Strengthens and conditions your legs, buttocks, hips, back, shoulders, and arms
8	The Crow	Stretches and strengthens your inner thighs, pelvic girdle, legs, buttocks, upper torso, and arms; tones and conditions your abdomen and core
8	The Runner	Strengthens and tones your legs, buttocks, back, shoulders, and arms; enhances balance and coordination
8	The Rise and Shine	Enhances balance, coordination, and overall body toning and stretching
9	The Twister	Strengthens and tones your abdomen, sides, and back; opens up your upper torso and arms
9	The Plow	Strengthens and conditions your core, abdomen, back, and legs; stretches and tones your arms
10	The Lightning Bolt	Builds strength and brings flexibility to your legs, buttocks, hips, back, and shoulders
10	The Swimmer	Strengthens and tones your arms, back, buttocks, legs, and abdomen
11	The Tree	Strengthens your legs, core, trunk, upper torso, and arms; develops balance, coordination, and stability
11	The Dancer	Helps stretch your quads, back, and shoulder girdle; enhances balance and stability
11	The Straddle	Stretches your groin, hips, and legs; strengthens your abdomen, back, and biceps
12	The Flying Locust	Strengthens and tones the front and back of your body; strengthens your shoulders, arms, chest, legs, and buttocks
12	The Locust	Strengthens your shoulders, chest, arms, legs, buttocks, and abdominal muscles
12	The Staff	Strengthens your shoulders, chest, arms, legs, buttocks, and abdominal muscles
12	The Burning Boat	Strengthens your core and abdominal muscles; builds endurance and stamina
12	The Archer	Strengthens, stretches, and tones your back and legs

Volleyball

Volleyball, like basketball, exercises many different muscle groups because you move your body in so many different ways. The sport demands balance and agility, the ability to jumpstart your energy reserves when needed, and the lung capacity to keep going. But those are just the requirements to play seriously; to be a good volleyball player, you need strength, power, speed, and physical fitness along with the balance and coordination.

Injuries often occur to your hands, fingers, and wrists from contact with the ball. Because you jump so often, you're at risk of ankle injuries from landing unevenly from aerial positions. The exercises in Table 16-5 are designed to strengthen your ankles and the core muscles of your trunk to give you better balance and coordination.

Warm-up exercises (see Chapter 6): Big Shoulder Release, Backward Shoulder Roll, Forward Shoulder Roll, Side Bender, Wrist Rotator, Hip Twister, Quad Stretcher, All-Out Hamstring Stretcher

Table 16-5		A Volleyballer's Workout
Chapter	*Exercise*	*Notes*
7	The Mountain	Opens up your chest, back, and spine; increases your shoulders' and arms' range of motion; enhances balance, coordination, and stability
7	Heaven and Earth	Stretches and lengthens your back, sides, arms, and legs
7	The Rag Doll	Releases tension in your head, neck, shoulders, and back; conditions your abdominal muscles, back, and legs
7	The Airplane	Strengthens and conditions your legs, back, and arms; enhances balance and stability
7	The Warrior II	Strengthens and conditions your legs, the core muscles of your trunk, your torso, shoulders, and arms
7	The Camel	Opens up your chest; strengthens your shoulders, arms, and legs; brings flexibility to your shoulders
7	The Dog	Offers total-body strengthening and conditioning

Chapter	Exercise	Notes
7	The Frog	Stretches your groin, hips, and pelvic girdle; stretches and strengthens your legs
8	The Chair	Strengthens and conditions your legs, buttocks, hips, back, shoulders, and arms
8	The Skater	Strengthens and conditions your hips, buttocks, abdomen, back, and legs
8	The Crow	Stretches and strengthens your inner thighs, pelvic girdle, legs, buttocks, upper torso, and arms; tones and conditions your abdomen and core
8	The Runner	Strengthens and tones your legs, buttocks, back, shoulders, and arms; enhances balance and coordination
8	The Rise and Shine	Enhances balance, coordination, and overall body tone and flexibility
9	The Pigeon	Stretches your legs, groin, inner thighs, hips, and pelvic girdle; tones your arms and biceps
10	The Lightning Bolt	Builds strength and brings flexibility to your legs, buttocks, hips, back, and shoulders
10	The Half Moon	Offers balance, stability, and strength for your entire body
10	The Swimmer	Strengthens and tones your arms, back, buttocks, legs, and abdomen
10	The Dolphin	Strengthens and conditions your upper torso, arms, abdomen, back, and legs; stretches your back and legs
11	The Horse	Strengthens and tones your abdomen, arms, back, buttocks, and legs
11	The Tree	Strengthens your legs, core, trunk, upper torso, and arms; develops balance, coordination, and stability
11	The Dancer	Helps stretch your quads, back, and shoulder girdle; enhances balance and stability

(continued)

Chapter	Exercise	Notes
	Table 16-5 *(continued)*	
11	The Eagle	Strengthens your core, legs, buttocks, abdomen, back, shoulders, and arms; develops balance, coordination, focus, and concentration
12	The Cow to Cat	Stretches and tones your back and spine; conditions your abdomen, legs, and buttocks
12	The Flying Locust	Strengthens and tones the front and back of your body; strengthens your shoulders, arms, chest, legs, and buttocks
12	The Locust	Strengthens your shoulders, chest, arms, legs, buttocks, and abdominal muscles
12	The Staff	Strengthens your shoulders, chest, arms, legs, buttocks, and abdominal muscles
12	The Burning Boat	Strengthens your core abdominal muscles; builds endurance
12	The Archer	Strengthens your core muscles; stretches and tones your back and legs

Power Walking (and Power Breathing)

Power walking isn't something new under the sun, but fitness experts and health-conscious people have recently taken a new interest in the activity because its health results are so apparent and so quickly achieved (Chapter 6 describes some of the health benefits of walking).

Your hip, buttock, and leg muscles get a workout during a power walk. As a power walker, you need to condition your upper torso so you can balance better as you walk. The exercises in Table 16-6 are designed to tone, condition, strengthen, and stretch your legs and upper torso. They also create a greater range of movement for your hips and legs.

Warm-up exercises (see Chapter 6): Side Bender, Hip Twister, Quad Stretcher, All-Out Hamstring Stretcher

Table 16-6		A Power Walker's Workout
Chapter	*Exercise*	*Notes*
7	Heaven and Earth	Stretches and lengthens your back, sides, arms, and legs
7	The Rag Doll	Releases tension in your head, neck, shoulders, and back; conditions your abdominal muscles, back, and legs
7	The Exalted Warrior	Strengthens and conditions your legs, buttocks, back, shoulders, and arms; enhances balance and stability
7	The Warrior II	Strengthens and conditions your legs, the core muscles of your trunk and torso, and your shoulders and arms
7	The Camel	Opens up your chest; strengthens your shoulders, arms, and legs; brings flexibility to your shoulders
7	The Dog	Offers total-body strengthening and conditioning
7	The Frog	Stretches your groin, hips, and pelvic girdle; stretches and strengthens your legs
8	The Chair	Strengthens and conditions your legs, buttocks, hips, back, shoulders, and arms
8	The Skater	Strengthens and conditions your hips, legs, buttocks, abdomen, back, and arms
8	The Crow	Stretches and strengthens your inner thighs, pelvic girdle, legs, buttocks, upper torso, and arms; tones and conditions your abdomen and core
8	The Rise and Shine	Enhances balance, coordination, and overall body tone and flexibility
9	The Twister	Strengthens and tones your abdomen, sides, and back; opens up your upper torso, chest, and arms
9	The Pigeon	Stretches your legs, groin, inner thighs, hips, and pelvic girdle; tones your arms and biceps
10	The Lightning Bolt	Builds strength and brings flexibility to your legs, buttocks, hips, back, and shoulders

(continued)

Table 16-6 *(continued)*

Chapter	Exercise	Notes
10	The Crescent Moon	Develops balance and coordination; stretches, strengthens, and conditions your legs, hips, buttocks, back, and groin
10	The Swimmer	Strengthens and tones your arms, back, buttocks, legs, and abdomen
10	The Dolphin	Strengthens and conditions your upper torso, arms, abdomen, back, and legs; stretches your back and legs
11	The Tree	Strengthens your legs, core, trunk, upper torso, and arms; develops balance, coordination, and stability
11	The Dancer	Stretches your quads, back, and shoulder girdle; enhances balance and stability
11	The Road Runner	Strengthens and conditions your hamstrings, legs, abdomen, back, and arms; enhances endurance and coordination
11	The Horse	Offers overall core body strengthening and conditioning
11	The Straddle	Stretches your groin, hips, and legs; strengthens your abdomen, back, and biceps
12	The Cow to Cat	Stretches and tones your back and spine; conditions your abdomen, legs, and buttocks
12	The Flying Locust	Strengthens and tones the front and back of your body; strengthens your shoulders, arms, chest, legs, and buttocks
12	The Locust	Strengthens and conditions your shoulders, chest, arms, legs, back, buttocks, and abdomen
12	The Staff	Strengthens your shoulders, chest, arms, legs, buttocks, and abdominal muscles
12	The Burning Boat	Strengthens your core abdominal muscles; builds endurance and stamina
12	The Archer	Strengthens your core muscles; stretches and tones your back and legs
12	The Belly Dancer	Strengthens and tones your hips, legs, and abdomen; brings flexibility to your hips and pelvis

Racket Sports

Racket sports such as tennis, squash, racquetball, badminton, and handball can be very demanding on your body. Players need flexibility, aerobic fitness, strength, stamina, and good hand-eye coordination. Racket sports involve short bursts of energy, lateral movement, sprinting, jumping, and arm swinging.

Having strong core muscles in your trunk and torso can greatly improve the power behind your movement — particularly your serves and returns of the ball or shuttlecock. In racket sports, you often have to reach beyond the norm to get to the ball or gracefully extend an arm to serve. By keeping your body supple and flexible, you can extend your arms and play your favorite sport for many years to come. The exercises in Table 16-7 can help balance your body and develop a greater range of motion in your swing.

Warm-up exercises (see Chapter 6): Side Bender, Hip Twister, Quad Stretcher, All-Out Hamstring Stretcher, The Big Stretcher

Table 16-7		A Racket-Sports Workout
Chapter	*Exercise*	*Notes*
7	The Mountain	Opens up your chest, back and spine; increases your shoulders' and arms' range of motion; enhances balance, coordination, and stability
7	Heaven and Earth	Stretches and lengthens your back, sides, arms, and legs
7	The Rag Doll	Releases tension in your head, neck, shoulders, and back; conditions your abdominal muscles, back, and legs
7	The Camel	Opens up your chest; strengthens your shoulders, arms, and legs; brings flexibility to your shoulders
7	The Dog	Offers total-body strengthening and conditioning
7	The Frog	Stretches your groin, hips, and pelvic girdle; stretches and strengthens your legs
8	The Chair	Strengthens and conditions your legs, buttocks, hips, back, shoulders, and arms
8	The Skater	Strengthens and conditions your hips, legs, buttocks, abdomen, back, and arms

(continued)

Table 16-7 *(continued)*

Chapter	Exercise	Notes
8	The Crow	Stretches and strengthens your inner thighs, pelvic girdle, legs, buttocks, upper torso, and arms; tones and conditions your abdomen and core
8	The Runner	Strengthens and tones your legs, buttocks, back, shoulders, and arms; enhances balance and coordination
8	The Eye of the Needle	Brings flexibility to your shoulders and back
8	The Rise and Shine	Enhances balance, coordination, and overall body tone and flexibility
9	The Sphinx	Strengthens and tones your upper back, shoulders, and arms; gently stretches your quads; conditions your buttocks
10	The Lightning Bolt	Strengthens and loosens your legs, buttocks, hips, back, and shoulders
10	The Crescent Moon	Develops balance and coordination; stretches, strengthens, and conditions your legs, hips, buttocks, back, and groin
10	The Dog to Plank	Strengthens and conditions your whole body
10	The Swimmer	Strengthens and tones your arms, back, buttocks, legs, and abdomen
10	The Lift	Strengthens your arms, back, abdomen, buttocks, and legs
11	The Tree	Strengthens your legs, core, trunk, upper torso, and arms; develops balance and coordination
11	The Dancer	Stretches your quads, back, and shoulder girdle; enhances balance and stability
11	The Russian Dancer	Develops balance and coordination; strengthens your legs, buttocks, abdomen, back, and arms; makes your hips more flexible
11	The Press	Stretches and strengthens your legs, groin, abdomen, back, shoulders, and arms
11	The Straddle	Stretches your groin, hips, and legs; strengthens your abdomen, back, and biceps

Chapter	Exercise	Notes
11	The Recharge	Opens up your groin, hips, and pelvic girdle; stretches your inner thighs
12	The Flying Locust	Strengthens and tones the front and back of your body; strengthens your shoulders, arms, chest, legs, and buttocks
12	The Locust	Strengthens and conditions your shoulders, chest, arms, legs, back, buttocks, and abdomen
12	The Love Handler	Stretches and conditions your groin, hips, and inner thighs; tones and conditions your sides and abdomen
12	The Staff	Strengthens your shoulders, chest, arms, legs, buttocks, and abdominal muscles
12	The Belly Crunch	Strengthens the muscles of your abdomen; lengthens and conditions your upper torso and sides

Golf

Golf is one of the most popular sports in the world. It teaches focus and concentration. And as long as you don't get mad at your own play, it teaches you a lesson similar to that taught by yoga — that relaxing can increase your powers of concentration. If you get serious about the sport, you soon notice the constant struggle between the conscious mind — analyzing, alert, and logical — and the subconscious mind — the well of inner knowing that's wakeful, present, and clear. Golfers who don't learn the nuances of the mental game remain frustrated or give up before mastering the sport. One of the biggest advantages golf has over other sports is that you play outdoors in a clean, healthy environment. Of course, golf is also a great social game when you play it with friends, family members, or business associates.

The exercises in Table 16-8 enhance your range of motion in the most important areas of your golf swing — such as your hips and shoulders. They also develop your ability to concentrate and focus, both of which are essential in golf.

Warm-up exercises (see Chapter 6): Side Bender, Hip Twister, Quad Stretcher, All-Out Hamstring Stretcher, The Big Stretcher

Table 16-8		A Golfer's Workout
Chapter	*Exercise*	*Notes*
7	The Mountain	Opens up your chest, back, and spine; increases your shoulders' and arms' range of motion; enhances balance, coordination, and stability
7	Heaven and Earth	Stretches and lengthens your back, sides, arms, and legs
7	The Rag Doll	Releases tension in your head, neck, shoulders, and back; conditions your abdominal muscles, back, and legs
7	The Airplane	Strengthens and conditions your legs, back, and arms; enhances balance and stability
7	The Triangle	Strengthens, stretches, and conditions your legs, hips, back, abdominal muscles, shoulders, and arms
7	The Exalted Warrior	Strengthens and conditions your legs, buttocks, back, shoulders, and arms; enhances balance and stability
7	The Warrior II	Strengthens and conditions your hips, legs, buttocks, abdomen, and back
7	The Camel	Opens up your chest; strengthens your shoulders, arms, and legs; adds flexibility to your shoulders
7	The Table	Strengthens and conditions your trunk, abdomen, arms, buttocks, and legs
7	The Cat	Stretches your back, spine, neck, and shoulders; strengthens and conditions your back, abdomen, buttocks, and legs
7	The Dog	Offers total-body strengthening and conditioning
7	The Bridge	Stretches and conditions your trunk, legs, buttocks, abdomen, arms, and shoulders
7	The Frog	Stretches your groin, hips, and pelvic girdle; stretches and strengthens your legs
7	The Zen	Reduces stress; improves your breathing technique; clears your mind; increases focus and concentration

Chapter	Exercise	Notes
8	The Chair	Strengthens and conditions your legs, buttocks, hips, back, shoulders, and arms
8	The Skater	Strengthens and conditions your hips, legs, buttocks, abdomen, back, and arms
8	The Runner	Strengthens and tones your legs, buttocks, back, shoulders, and arms; enhances balance and coordination
8	The Eye of the Needle	Brings flexibility to your shoulders and back
8	The Twisted Triangle	Stretches and strengthens your legs, hips, pelvis, back, and sides; tones and conditions your abdomen and arms; develops balance and coordination
8	The Rise and Shine	Stretches and strengthens your legs, hips, pelvis, back, and sides; tones and conditions your abdomen and arms; develops balance and coordination
9	The Twister	Strengthens and tones your abdomen, sides, and back; opens up your upper torso, chest, and arms
9	The Child's Pose	Stretches your inner thighs, quads, hips, groin, and back; tones and conditions your back, shoulders, and arms
9	The Lion	Opens up your inner thighs, groin, hips, and pelvic girdle; strengthens and conditions your back and abdomen; releases stress
10	The Crescent Moon	Develops balance and coordination; stretches, strengthens, and conditions your legs, hips, buttocks, back, and groin
10	The Half Moon	Conditions and strengthens your back, arms, and the core muscles of your trunk and torso
10	The Swimmer	Strengthens and tones your arms, back, buttocks, legs, and abdomen
10	The Lift	Strengthens your arms, back, abdomen, buttocks, and legs
10	The Side Plank	Strengthens your trunk, abdomen, arms, legs, sides, and buttocks

(continued)

Table 16-8 *(continued)*

Chapter	Exercise	Notes
11	The Tree	Strengthens your legs, core, trunk, upper torso, and arms; promotes balance, coordination, and stability
11	The Dancer	Stretches your quads, back, and shoulder girdle; enhances balance and stability
11	The Eagle	Strengthens your core, legs, buttocks, abdomen, back, shoulders, and arms; develops balance, coordination, focus, and concentration
11	The Russian Dancer	Strengthens your legs, buttocks, abdomen, back, shoulders, and arms; develops balance, coordination, focus, and concentration
11	The Side Bow	Strengthens and conditions your hips, thighs, buttocks, abdomen, arms, and sides; stretches the front of your body
11	The Horse	Offers total-body strengthening and conditioning
12	The Cow to Cat	Stretches and tones your back and spine; conditions your abdomen, legs, and buttocks
12	The Flying Locust	Strengthens and tones the front and back of your body; strengthens your shoulders, arms, chest, legs, and buttocks
12	The Locust	Strengthens and conditions your shoulders, chest, arms, legs, back, buttocks, and abdomen
12	The Love Handler	Stretches and conditions your groin, hips, and inner thighs; tones and conditions your sides and abdomen
12	The Staff	Strengthens your shoulders, chest, arms, legs, buttocks, and abdominal muscles
12	The Archer	Strengthens the core of your body; stretches and tones your back and legs
12	The Belly Dancer	Strengthens and tones your hips, legs, and abdomen; brings flexibility to your hips and pelvis

Skiing

Skiing requires dexterity, balance, and the ability to concentrate — qualities you can develop through yoga-with-weights exercises. Yoga with weights builds strength and improves body awareness, balance, and flexibility.

As far as skiing is concerned, one of the biggest benefits of yoga with weights is the attention to breathing. You're safer when you're in a relaxed and aware state. The attention yoga-with-weights exercises pay to breathing will develop steadiness of mind so you can be fully in the moment as you ski, and that, in turn, helps prevent injuries.

Skiing taxes the muscles of your lower body. The exercises in Table 16-9 build the muscles in your lower body and make your hips and quads more flexible and your knees stronger. Because range of motion is so vital for quick response times when you're skiing, we also include exercises that increase the range of motion in your legs and arms. These exercises awaken new sources of joy and exhilaration that you can take to the slopes.

Warm-up exercises (see Chapter 6): Forward Shoulder Roll, Backward Shoulder Roll, Quad Stretcher, All-Out Hamstring Stretcher

Table 16-9		A Skier's Workout
Chapter	*Exercise*	*Notes*
7	The Rag Doll	Stretches out your legs, back, head, neck, shoulders, and arms
7	The Warrior II	Strengthens your legs, buttocks, trunk, and upper torso
7	The Dog	Offers total-body strengthening and conditioning
7	The Frog	Opens up your groin, hips, and pelvis; stretches and strengthens your legs
8	The Skater	Strengthens and tones your legs, buttocks, abdomen, back, shoulders, and arms; enhances balance and stability
8	The Runner	Strengthens and tones your legs, buttocks, back, shoulders, and arms; enhances balance and coordination

(continued)

Table 16-9 *(continued)*

Chapter	Exercise	Notes
8	The Warrior I	Strengthens and tones your legs, buttocks, back, shoulders, and arms; opens up your hips and groin
8	The Rise and Shine	Strengthens and stretches your legs, back, shoulders, and arms; enhances fluidity of movement
9	The Twister	Strengthens and tones your abdomen, sides, and back; opens up your upper chest; stretches your arms
9	The Pigeon	Stretches your hips and groin
9	The Plow	Tones and strengthens your core muscles, legs, and back
10	The Swimmer	Strengthens and tones your arms, back, buttocks, legs, and abdomen
10	The Lightning Bolt	Stretches and tones your arms, back, sides, and legs; enhances balance and stability
11	The Straddle	Stretches your groin, hips, and legs; strengthens your abdomen, back, and biceps
11	The Road Runner	Stretches and strengthens your hamstrings, back, and arms; tones your abdomen; enhances coordination
11	The Dancer	Stretches and tones your quadriceps and back; conditions your shoulder girdle, arms, and abdomen; develops balance and stability
12	The Cow to Cat	Opens up your back and spine; strengthens and tones your abdomen, legs, buttocks, and core
12	The Love Handler	Stretches your pelvic girdle and legs; tones and conditions your abdomen and sides
12	The Burning Boat	Strengthens and conditions your abdomen, arms, legs, and back
12	The Archer	Strengthens your core; stretches and tones your back and legs

Football and Soccer

Football and soccer (or American football and football, depending on your loyalties) require stamina, physical strength, quickness, and the ability to concentrate in spite of fatigue and exhaustion. Both sports make extraordinary demands on the muscles of your legs, and football — especially if you play on the offensive or defensive line — requires great upper-body strength as well. On account of the physical demands and the variety of body movements, football and soccer players are more prone to injury than athletes in other sports.

Yoga with weights can help prevent injuries and improve performance because it increases your agility and flexibility. It enables you to move with a greater range of motion, which gives you the freedom and confidence to be a better player. Baron Baptiste, Sherri's brother and a renowned yoga teacher, served as the "peak performance specialist" for the Philadelphia Eagles professional football team for five years in the 1990s. Under his yoga tutelage, the number of injuries on the team dropped significantly; Baron credits yoga for this development.

The exercises we recommend in Table 16-10 require you to work major and minor muscle groups simultaneously. These exercises help you improve your overall fitness, rehabilitate injuries, and prolong your football and soccer playing days.

Warm-up exercises (see Chapter 6): Forward Shoulder Roll, Backward Shoulder Roll, Quad Stretcher, All-Out Hamstring Stretcher

Table 16-10		A Footballer's Workout
Chapter	*Exercise*	*Notes*
7	The Rag Doll	Stretches out your legs, back, head, neck, shoulders, and arms
7	The Warrior II	Strengthens your legs, buttocks, trunk, and upper torso
7	The Dog	Offers total-body strengthening and conditioning
7	The Frog	Opens up your groin, hips, and pelvis; stretches and strengthens your legs
8	The Skater	Strengthens and tones your legs, buttocks, abdomen, back, shoulders, and arms; enhances balance and stability

(continued)

Table 16-10 *(continued)*

Chapter	Exercise	Notes
8	The Runner	Strengthens and tones your legs, buttocks, back, shoulders, and arms; enhances balance and coordination
8	The Warrior I	Strengthens and tones your legs, buttocks, back, shoulders, and arms; opens up your hips and groin
8	The Rise and Shine	Strengthens and stretches your legs, back, shoulders, and arms; enhances fluidity of movement
9	The Twister	Strengthens and tones your abdomen, sides, and back; opens up your upper chest; stretches your arms
9	The Pigeon	Stretches your hips and groin
9	The Plow	Tones and strengthens your core muscles, legs, and back
10	The Swimmer	Strengthens and tones your arms, back, buttocks, legs, and abdomen
10	The Lightning Bolt	Stretches and tones your arms, back, sides, and legs; enhances balance and stability
11	The Straddle	Stretches your groin, hips, and legs; strengthens your abdomen, back, and biceps
11	The Road Runner	Stretches and strengthens your hamstrings, back, and arms; tones your abdomen; enhances coordination
11	The Dancer	Stretches and tones your quadriceps and back; conditions your shoulder girdle, arms, and abdomen; develops balance and stability
12	The Cow to Cat	Opens up your back and spine; strengthens and tones your abdomen, legs, buttocks, and core
12	The Love Handler	Stretches your pelvic girdle and legs; tones and conditions your abdomen and sides
12	The Burning Boat	Strengthens and conditions your abdomen, arms, legs, and back
12	The Archer	Strengthens your core; stretches and tones your back and legs

Baseball and Softball

Baseball and softball can be very demanding because they require short bursts of energy, focus and concentration, good hand-eye coordination, side-to-side movement, and arm strength.

The yoga-with-weights exercises in Table 16-11 can help bring muscle balance to your body and develop a greater range for your swing and your throwing motions.

Warm-up exercises (see Chapter 6): Side Bender, Hip Twister, Quad Stretcher, All-Out Hamstring Stretcher, The Big Stretcher

Table 16-11		A Ballplayer's Workout
Chapter	*Exercise*	*Notes*
7	The Mountain	Opens up your chest, back, and spine; increases your shoulders' and arms' range of motion; enhances balance, coordination, and stability
7	Heaven and Earth	Stretches and lengthens your back, sides, arms, and legs
7	The Rag Doll	Releases tension in your head, neck, shoulders, and back; conditions your abdominal muscles, back, and legs
7	The Camel	Opens up your chest; strengthens your shoulders, arms, and legs; brings flexibility to your shoulders
7	The Dog	Offers total-body strengthening and conditioning
7	The Frog	Stretches your groin, hips, and pelvic girdle; stretches and strengthens your legs
8	The Chair	Strengthens and conditions your legs, buttocks, hips, back, shoulders, and arms
8	The Skater	Strengthens and conditions your hips, legs, buttocks, abdomen, back, and arms
8	The Crow	Stretches and strengthens your inner thighs, pelvic girdle, legs, buttocks, upper torso, and arms; tones and conditions your abdomen and core

(continued)

Table 16-11 *(continued)*

Chapter	Exercise	Notes
8	The Runner	Strengthens and tones your legs, buttocks, back, shoulders, and arms; enhances balance and coordination
8	The Eye of the Needle	Brings flexibility to your shoulders and back
8	The Rise and Shine	Enhances balance, coordination, and overall body toning and stretching
9	The Sphinx	Strengthens and tones your upper back, shoulders, and arms; gently stretches your quads; conditions your buttocks
10	The Lightning Bolt	Strengthens and loosens your legs, buttocks, hips, back, and shoulders
10	The Crescent Moon	Develops balance and coordination; stretches, strengthens, and conditions your legs, hips, buttocks, back, and groin
10	The Dog to Plank	Strengthens and conditions your whole body
10	The Swimmer	Strengthens and tones your arms, back, buttocks, legs, and abdomen
10	The Lift	Strengthens your arms, back, abdomen, buttocks, and legs
11	The Tree	Strengthens your legs, core, trunk, upper torso, and arms; develops balance, coordination, and stability
11	The Dancer	Stretches your quads, back, and shoulder girdle; enhances balance and stability
11	The Russian Dancer	Develops balance, stability, and coordination; strengthens your legs, buttocks, abdomen, back, and arms; makes your hips more flexible
11	The Press	Stretches and strengthens your legs, groin, abdomen, back, shoulders, and arms
11	The Straddle	Stretches your groin, hips, and legs; strengthens your abdomen, back, and biceps
11	The Recharge	Opens up your groin, hips, and pelvic girdle; stretches your inner thighs

Chapter	Exercise	Notes
12	The Flying Locust	Strengthens and tones the front and back of your body; strengthens your shoulders, arms, chest, legs, and buttocks
12	The Locust	Strengthens and conditions your shoulders, chest, arms, legs, back, buttocks, and abdomen
12	The Love Handler	Stretches and conditions your groin, hips, and inner thighs; tones and conditions your sides and abdomen
12	The Staff	Strengthens your shoulders, chest, arms, legs, buttocks, and abdominal muscles
12	The Belly Crunch	Strengthens the muscles of your abdomen; lengthens and conditions your upper torso and sides

Cross-Training

Cross-training refers to a training routine in which you engage in several different forms of exercise each week. Instead of engaging, for example, in weightlifting three times a week, you lift weights, run, and play basketball. The idea behind cross-training is to exercise your entire body.

Yoga with weights is, in and of itself, something of a cross-training exercise program because it works so many muscle groups and tests your balancing and endurance skills. It's a great low-impact way to cross-train. Yoga with weights strengthens your cardiovascular system, bones, muscles, and joints; reduces your body fat; and improves your flexibility, balance, and coordination. Table 16-12 presents a "greatest-hits" list of yoga-with-weights exercises for cross-trainers.

Warm-up exercises (see Chapter 6): Chin-Chest Tuck, Head Turner, Lateral Neck Release, Backward Shoulder Roll, Forward Shoulder Roll, Hip Twister, Quad Stretcher, All-Out Hamstring Stretcher, The Big Stretcher

Chapter	Exercise	Notes
	Table 16-12	**A Cross-Trainer's Workout**
7	The Mountain	Opens up your chest, back, and spine; increases your shoulders' and arms' range of motion; develops balance, coordination, and stability
7	Heaven and Earth	Stretches and lengthens your back, sides, arms, and legs
7	The Rag Doll	Releases tension in your head, neck, shoulders, and back; conditions your abdominal muscles, back, and legs
7	The Airplane	Strengthens and conditions your legs, back, and arms; develops balance and stability
7	The Triangle	Strengthens, stretches, and conditions your legs, hips, back, abdominal muscles, shoulders, and arms
7	The Exalted Warrior	Strengthens and conditions your legs, buttocks, back, shoulders, and arms; enhances balance and stability
7	The Dog	Offers total-body strengthening and conditioning
7	The Bridge	Stretches and conditions your trunk, legs, buttocks, abdomen, arms, and shoulders
7	The Frog	Stretches your groin, hips, and pelvic girdle; stretches and strengthens your legs
8	The Chair	Strengthens and conditions your legs, buttocks, hips, back, shoulders, and arms
8	The Crow	Stretches and strengthens your inner thighs, pelvic girdle, legs, buttocks, upper torso, and arms; tones and conditions your abdomen and core
8	The Runner	Strengthens and tones your legs, buttocks, back, shoulders, and arms; enhances balance and coordination
8	The Eye of the Needle	Brings flexibility to your shoulders and back
8	The Twisted Triangle	Stretches and strengthens your legs, hips, pelvis, back, and sides; tones and conditions your abdomen and arms; develops balance and coordination

Chapter	Exercise	Notes
8	The Rise and Shine	Stretches and strengthens your legs, hips, pelvis, back, and sides; tones and conditions your abdomen and arms; develops balance and coordination
9	The Twister	Strengthens and tones your abdomen, sides, and back; opens up your upper torso, chest, and arms
9	The Pigeon	Stretches your legs, groin, inner thighs, hips, and pelvic girdle; tones your biceps
9	The Plow	Strengthens and conditions your abdomen, upper and lower torso, legs, and buttocks
10	The Crescent Moon	Develops balance and coordination; stretches, strengthens, and conditions your legs, hips, buttocks, back, and groin
10	The Dog to Plank	Strengthens and conditions your entire body
10	The Side Plank	Strengthens your trunk, abdomen, arms, legs, sides, and buttocks
10	The Swimmer	Strengthens and tones your arms, back, buttocks, legs, and abdomen
10	The Dolphin	Strengthens and conditions your upper torso, arms, abdomen, back, and legs; stretches your back and legs
10	The Lift	Strengthens your arms, back, abdomen, buttocks, and legs
11	The Tree	Strengthens your legs, core, trunk, upper torso, and arms; develops balance and coordination
11	The Dancer	Stretches your quads, back, and shoulder girdle; enhances balance and stability
11	The Eagle	Strengthens your core, legs, buttocks, abdomen, back, shoulders, and arms; develops balance, coordination, focus, and concentration
11	The Side Bow	Strengthens and conditions your hips, thighs, buttocks, abdomen, arms, and sides; stretches the front of your body

(continued)

Table 16-12 *(continued)*

Chapter	Exercise	Notes
11	The Horse	Strengthens and conditions the core of your body
11	The Straddle	Stretches your groin, hips, and legs; strengthens your abdomen, back, and biceps
12	The Cow to Cat	Stretches and tones your back and spine; conditions your abdomen, legs, and buttocks
12	The Flying Locust	Strengthens and tones the front and back of your body; strengthens your shoulders, arms, chest, legs, and buttocks
12	The Locust	Strengthens and conditions your shoulders, chest, arms, legs, back, buttocks, and abdomen
12	The Love Handler	Stretches and conditions your groin, hips, and inner thighs; tones and conditions your sides and abdomen
12	The Staff	Strengthens your shoulders, chest, arms, legs, buttocks, and abdominal muscles
12	The Burning Boat	Strengthens and conditions your abdomen, arms, legs, and back
12	The Belly Crunch	Strengthens your trunk, abdomen, upper torso, and sides

Chapter 17

Girl Talk

*T*his chapter looks into how yoga with weights can address issues of health and well-being specific to women — premenstrual syndrome, maintaining bone density, mid-life depression, graceful aging, and childbirth. We even offer a handful of yoga-with-weights exercises designed especially for pregnant women.

This chapter may be called "Girl Talk," but that doesn't mean male readers can't eavesdrop. In fact, we encourage men to read this chapter, because they can discover plenty about the women in their lives: who they really are, how to cherish them, and how to make them happy.

Addressing Women's Health Issues through Yoga with Weights

Yoga with weights has some important advantages for women. The exercises tend to increase bone density and ease the symptoms of premenstrual syndrome. They even help in fighting depression and preparing for childbirth. Don't believe us? You'd better keep reading.

Increasing bone density

Because the ovarian hormone estrogen plays an important part in maintaining strong bones, and because a woman's production of estrogen decreases when she reaches menopause, women (more so than men) lose bone density as they grow older. *Bone density* is a measure of how tightly packed the cells and molecules in a bone are. The higher the bone density, the less likely a bone is to fracture or break, and the faster it can heal.

Bone density reaches its peak when women are between the ages of 30 and 35, and then it begins to decline as estrogen production decreases. Most losses in bone density occur when women are in their 40s, during the onset of premenopause; at about age 40, men and women usually experience loss of bone density because they don't exercise as often. Diet plays a key role, too, because older people can't absorb the calcium in their food as readily. Today, many doctors test the bone density of women when they're in their mid 30s to 40s to establish a baseline for bone density loss.

By exercising and eating right, *premenopausal* (before menopause) and *perimenopausal* (in the menopausal stage) women can build strong bones during their 20s and early 30s and then maintain strong bones from about age 35 onward.

Yoga with weights can help you maintain bone density because your body builds strong bones under the stress of exercise. As you lift weights and your muscles pull against your bones, your body reacts by making the cells in your bones stronger and denser to support the pull of your muscles. For example, when you do arm curls, the bones in your upper arms gain bone density. Yoga-with-weights exercises are excellent for women because they help offset the loss of bone density that comes with menopause and aging.

Fighting depression

Depression can creep into the life of a woman at any time. Puberty, young motherhood, starting a career, an empty nest, and menopause all cause peculiar kinds of stress; and all can cause depression. Many women come into our yoga classes with the idea of treating the symptoms of common depression. These women want to return a sense of balance to their lives. Most get a welcome boost of energy from yoga with weights, as well as a reduction of stress in their lives.

Yoga with weights, like all forms of exercise, releases *endorphins* in your body — the natural feel-good chemicals that give you a sense of well-being (the Greek root for the word endorphin is the same as the root for morphine). Exercising helps you sleep better, and sleep and endorphins are natural antidotes for depression.

Yoga with weights also helps combat depression because the attention you pay to breathing opens up your chest and allows your lungs to fill with life-giving oxygen. This improves your circulation and opens up your heart, so to speak, making you feel happier. Stop what you're doing right now, just for a moment, and take a deep breath. Do you feel a "big smile on your chest?"

Handling premenstrual syndrome

By some estimates, four in ten women and as many as 70 to 90 percent of women of childbearing age have premenstrual syndrome, or PMS. A balanced, nutritional diet and proper amounts of exercise may be the keys to reducing PMS symptoms. Yoga with weights can help lesson the symptoms because the squatting exercises deliver more blood to your pelvic floor, the endorphins released during the exercises combat depression, and the breathing techniques help you to relax and de-stress. (Be sure to read Chapter 13 to address your diet.)

A Special Workout for Expecting Mothers

Whatever decision you make about how you want to give birth, yoga-with-weights exercises can gently help you prepare for the big event by making you stronger and increasing your ability to focus and concentrate. In addition, the exercises help you maintain a high energy level after the baby is born and help you get back into shape.

The exercises we present here are designed to help prepare pregnant women for labor and condition them mentally and emotionally for giving birth. Even if you walk for only a few minutes every day and adopt the breathing and mindfulness techniques you find in this book (see Chapters 4 and 5), you'll feel and look your best during and after your pregnancy. The yoga-with-weights exercises in this chapter help strengthen your back, make you comfortable while you're pregnant, and prepare your pelvic floor for a healthy delivery when the time comes to give birth. Use the last exercise as an affirmation to plant the seeds of well-being and make yours a joyous childbirth.

Before beginning any new exercise program, pregnant women should consult with a health professional or primary prenatal care physician, especially if they have pregnancy-induced high blood pressure, early contractions, or vaginal bleeding. The exercises we've designed for pregnant women are slow, comforting, and relaxing exercises. Nevertheless, exercising can pose risks to pregnant women, especially those in or beyond the sixth month of their pregnancies. In our experience, pregnant women who have permission from doctors to exercise have no trouble doing standing yoga-with-weights exercises and poses that require you to have the support of a chair. Starting at the sixth month, however, you may need to stop doing exercises that require lying on your belly or back. Twisting exercises also aren't recommended for pregnant women, so to be on the safe side, we don't offer twisting exercises in this chapter.

Yoga breathing and childbirth

Sherri Baptiste is the mother of four children. Here's what she says about yoga breathing and childbirth:

"I was always surprised to hear, while I was giving birth, that I have a high threshold for pain. What I really have is an understanding of the power of yoga breathing and an ability to harness that power. During labor, I was able to stay calm as the contractions intensified. I completed labor without the use of any drugs."

"Throughout labor, I felt that I had yoga breathing as a tool and a friend to help me in the challenge to stay calm and be present. Yoga breathing took the edge off as the waves of pain grew stronger and stronger with each contraction and the forces of labor took over. In each phase of delivery, the power of the breathing allowed me to draw my attention and all my strength into the moment and into what I was doing."

"I'm no hero or saint when it comes to pain. I felt it every inch of the way as those babies of mine — two daughters and two sons — worked their way out into the world. I was one of those women who didn't look forward to labor. I just wanted to get it over with as quickly, safely, and painlessly as possible — but without any drugs."

"I learned from giving birth that, realistically speaking, the mother is just along for the ride. You have little control over any of it. But you do have the power within yourself — breath by breath, moment by moment — to help nature direct your childbirth and support your ease and well-being. Yoga breathing can be your best friend, especially when you're giving birth. It can help you to better manage the pain of childbirth, harness the strength you need, and discover the timeless wisdom that every woman carries within herself to give birth and become a mother."

Exercise gently when you're pregnant. Notice any signals of discomfort, and stop doing an exercise if it doesn't feel right. You want your workout to gently relax your whole body, leaving you with a peaceful sense of well-being.

Be sure to read Chapter 4, which offers yoga breathing techniques. During childbirth, the power of the breathing (and the controlled state of mind that breathing can bring about) may help to slow down or speed up your labor as necessary. Breathing can help you smoothly ride out the waves of labor, which is why Lamaze and Bradley classes teach breathing techniques for expectant mothers. These breathing techniques train mothers to relax during delivery.

Courage and Strength

The purpose of Courage and Strength is to prepare you for childbirth by giving you the tools and techniques necessary to build your courage and strength. You have to remember that courage isn't the absence of fear, but the ability to proceed skillfully, moment by moment, with conviction and clarity.

This exercise helps train you to focus during childbirth, opening your heart and mind to the process at hand. It strengthens your back and spine and shows you how to open your pelvic area. It also strengthens your arms so you can carry your baby easily after you give birth. You're going to have to do plenty of multitasking: holding your baby, preparing the bottles, unloading grocery bags, and so on. It helps to have strong muscles!

Use the lightest hand weights you have for this exercise. Also, grab a blanket. Follow these steps to find your courage and strength:

1. **Sit on the floor with your right leg straight, your left foot next to the inner thigh of your right leg, and a folded blanket under your left knee.**

   If you're well along in your pregnancy, place your right leg to the side to comfortably accommodate your belly. You can also place a blanket behind your buttocks, as the model in Figure 17-1 has, for support in case you lose your balance.

2. **Pick up the weights and hold them at ear level or a bit higher with your elbows bent (see Figure 17-1a).**

   This is the starting position. Look straight ahead. How high you lift the weights depends on how high you can comfortably hold them.

3. **Inhaling to a count of four, lift your arms up (see Figure 17-1b).**

   Weightlifters call this a *shoulder press*. Don't strain; make sure you stop at a comfortable level.

4. **Exhaling to a count of four, lower your arms to the starting position (see Figure 17-1a).**

Figure 17-1: Strengthening your back and arms gives you courage during and after childbirth.

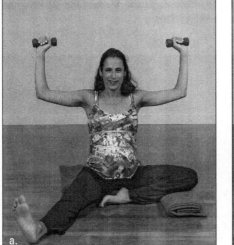 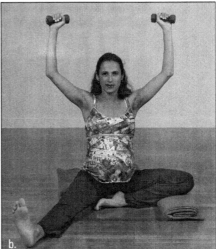

Repeat this exercise six to eight times, pause to rest for as long as you need, and then do six to eight more repetitions with your left leg straightened.

Opening the Way

Opening the Way is an exercise that helps to prepare your pelvic girdle for childbirth by opening your groin and supporting the relaxation and release in your pelvis. The *pelvic girdle* is the boney structure surrounding your pelvis. During vaginal childbirth, the baby passes through the opening in the pelvic girdle. The exercise also strengthens and tones your upper torso, including your back and spine, and teaches you to breathe fully by encouraging good posture. Breathing properly with good posture is a big help during childbirth, when comfort matters so much.

Grab your lightest hand weights and two folded blankets for this exercise. Follow these steps to open the way:

1. **Sit cross-legged on the floor with a folded blanket under each knee and your hands, holding the weights, resting on your knees with your palms facing upward (see Figure 17-2a).**

    This is the starting position. Look straight ahead.

2. **Inhaling to a count of four, bend your elbows (see Figure 17-2b).**

    Weightlifters call this a *bicep curl.* Feel your bicep muscles working. Make sure your elbows stay close to your ribs.

3. **Exhaling to a count of four, slowly lower the weights to the starting position (see Figure 17-2a).**

Repeat this exercise six to eight times, pause to rest for as long as you need, and then do six to eight more repetitions.

Figure 17-2:
Opening the Way widens your pelvic girdle and strengthens your spine.

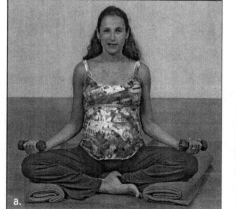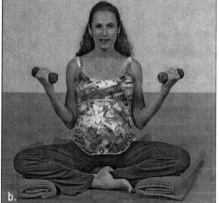

The Mother Goddess

The Mother Goddess helps prepare your pelvic girdle for childbirth by conditioning and toning the muscles surrounding it. The exercise also strengthens your legs, inner thighs, and back; conditions you to stay steady and balanced; and trains you to be able to breathe in a consistent way when the rigors of childbirth are challenging you.

You need hand weights for this exercise. If you're afraid of tipping over, you should grab a folded blanket as well, which you can put under your heels to give you more support when you squat (shown in Figure 17-3a). Follow these steps to complete the Mother Goddess exercise:

1. **Squat on the balls of your feet with your elbows against your knees and your hands joined in front of your chest (see Figure 17-3a).**

    This is the starting position. Keep your knees wide to accommodate your belly. Hold this position for three or four calm and steady breaths before proceeding.

    If you have trouble squatting and keeping your balance, do this exercise with your back against a wall, or sit on a low stool to start this exercise.

2. **Slowly inhaling to a count of four, pick up the hand weights, rise to your feet — keeping your knees slightly bent — and raise the weights above your head (see Figure 17-3b).**

    Widen your stance by a couple of inches to get into this position.

3. **As you continue to inhale, keep rising until your legs are straight (see Figure 17-3c).**

4. **Slowly exhaling to a count of four, gently and smoothly return to the starting position (see Figure 17-3a).**

    Spread your knees, pressing your tailbone gently downward as you squat down.

Repeat this gentle squat and rise six times, pausing to rest between each repetition, and then repeat the exercise, if desired, another six times.

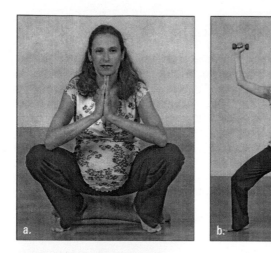

Figure 17-3:
The Mother
Goddess
prepares
you
physically
and
mentally for
childbirth.

Ending meditation: Divine Mother Affirmation

The purpose of the Divine Mother Affirmation is to center you and to teach you how to relax and calm your mind on your own. You're talking to yourself in a good way — like a coach sending the right message to be well and in harmony with it all. This practice isn't as much an exercise as it is a quiet meditation designed for expectant mothers.

You need three folded up blankets for this exercise. When you're ready, follow these steps to do the Divine Mother Affirmation:

1. **Sit cross-legged (or as near to cross-legged as you can) in a comfortable way, with one blanket under your buttocks and one under each knee.**

   You can sit with your back against a wall if doing so makes you more comfortable.

2. **Close your eyes and join your palms over your chest in a prayer pose (see Figure 17-4).**

3. **Quiet your mind and commune with yourself.**

   Quietly meditate for a moment on the life that's growing inside you. Listen to the gentle sound of your breathing. Silently repeat these words to yourself: "Breathing in, I calm body and mind, and breathing out, I smile; so be it." Feel free to pick your own words that take you to a state of greater well-being.

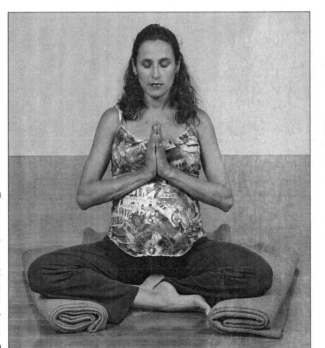

Figure 17-4:
The Divine Mother Affirmation is a quiet meditation for you and your baby alone.

Chapter 18

Exercises for Seniors

No matter your age, yoga-with-weights exercises can help you stay strong and supple. Therefore, we've designed the exercises in this chapter specifically for seniors. Here, you find a workout that emphasizes the importance of stretching, relaxing, and strengthening for promoting the general health and well-being of seniors. Still not convinced? Okay, the exercises also slow down and prevent premature aging!

You need a sturdy chair for the exercises in this chapter. The chair gives you confidence and makes you feel stable as you exercise so you can dive in without worrying about whether you'll lose your balance or fall. The chair should be short enough so you can sit on it without leaving your feet dangling. If you're short, you may need to place a footstool under your feet. The chair should have a strong back, because you need to grasp the back of the chair in some exercises.

To get the most from these exercises, maintain a concentrated focus on the alignment of your spine. Imagine or visualize your spine lengthening and realigning as you gently breathe in each exercise. We also ask you to take gentle, empowering, Complete Breaths as you do this workout (Chapter 4 looks into all aspects of breathing). Take your time not only with each exercise, but also with each inhale and exhale. Breathing is a barometer of how you're doing. If you're breathing too rapidly or holding your breath, you're probably working too hard, but if your breathing is steady and calm, you're probably working just right.

Use light weights to start. As you get stronger, gradually increase the size of the weights. Always work at your own level of ability and take into account the energy you have that day.

Reaping the Rewards of the Senior Workout

An old saying in the yoga tradition says that you're as youthful as your spine is supple and flexible. The exercises in this workout increase the strength and suppleness of your spine. It feels great to have a limber spine that's free to move in all directions, but a spine that moves with ease is important for safety reasons, too. For example, you'll be able to sit on the floor and get up without assistance, and you'll feel more youthful so you can do the physical activities that you really love.

The exercises in this workout also increase bone density. An excessive loss of bone density in the process of aging leaves your bones weakened and susceptible to fracturing and breaking. However, we have good news: Bone is living tissue, so it's in a constant state of regeneration. In a yoga-with-weights workout, your muscles have to work against the weights you carry, which puts stress on your bones and therefore increases bone density. You increase blood circulation to your muscles as well, which also builds bone density and muscle strength. You focus on keeping your body strong and upright, and you do exercises that are very gentle on your joints and connective tissues.

Along with building up your bone and muscle, the exercises in this chapter improve your coordination. Maintaining good coordination reduces your risk of falling and allows you to be more confident and sure of yourself.

People of all ages feel the natural urge to skip a workout now and then. In the case of seniors, however, the body needs more rest and repose on certain days, so you need to pay attention to those needs. But as much as you can, try to stay on track and do these exercises every other day. By consistently practicing these yoga-with-weights exercises, by paying attention to your breathing, and by following the meditation practices we describe in this book (see Chapter 6), you discover more physical freedom in your daily movements and in your life. You gain the confidence to be able to move with ease. When you begin to practice the exercises, you'll notice a greater level of mobility and strength. And the exercises help you maintain the strength and mobility that you already have, giving you healthy support for years to come.

Never force yourself or push too hard as you do this workout; use your experience to recognize when you should rest or press forward. The goal is to challenge yourself to do the exercises with a little more intensity and concentration each time you do them.

Candle Blowing

Candle Blowing warms you up for all the exercises in the senior yoga-with-weights workout. Although the exercise's name may conjure up images of cake, we call it Candle Blowing because we want you to focus on your breathing. Throughout the exercise, you breathe in and out with pursed lips as if you're blowing out the candles on a birthday cake. As you concentrate on your breathing and warming up your body, you work your bicep muscles and increase your blood circulation.

You need hand weights for this exercise. When you're ready to go, follow these steps:

1. **Sit in a chair with your elbows bent and the weights held at your thighs, palms facing upward (see Figure 18-1a).**

   This is the starting position. Sit upright with your shoulders squared, but don't allow your shoulders to creep up to your neck. Purse your lips for the proper breathing technique.

2. **Exhaling to a count of four, curl the weights to the level of your shoulders (see Figure 18-1b).**

   In weightlifting, this action is called a *bicep curl.* Pull your belly in, and use your belly as well as your arms to support the weights. Feel the air leave your lungs as you exhale.

3. **Inhaling to a count of four, lower the weights to the starting position (see Figure 18-1a).**

   Inhale slowly and deeply into your abdomen as you slowly lower the weights in rhythm with your breathing.

Repeat this exercise four to six times, pause to rest, and then do four to six more repetitions.

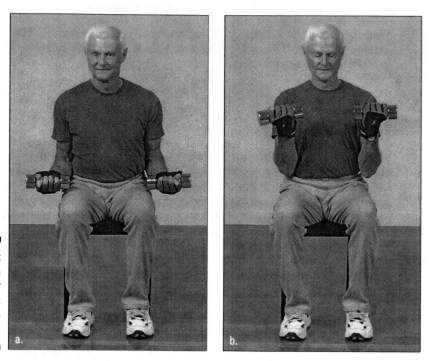

Figure 18-1:
Focus on
your
breathing as
you do
bicep curls.

The Mirror

The Mirror opens your chest and lungs, as well as the sides of your body, aiding in free breathing and improved flexibility. It also creates better range of motion in your neck and shoulders, making the exercise excellent for people who suffer from stiff necks and "frozen shoulders." Having more room to breathe deeply makes it easier to relax.

You need hand weights for this exercise. When you're ready, follow these steps:

1. **Sit in a chair with your elbows bent and the weights held at your thighs, palms facing upward, and fix your gaze on your right hand (see Figure 18-2a).**

   This is the starting position.

2. **Inhaling to a count of four, lift your right arm in a half-arc position until your hand is above your right shoulder, watching your right hand along the way (see Figure 18-2b).**

   Draw your belly in and up as you lift the weight, and reach only to a comfortable height. If you can, raise your hand straight up, as the model does in Figure 18-2. The goal it to reach as high as you can without forcing or straining.

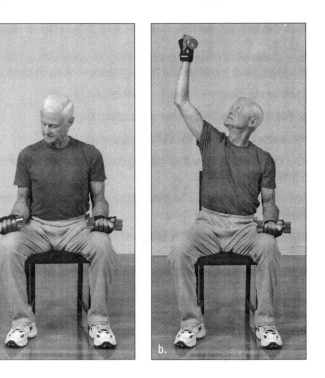

Figure 18-2:
Mirror,
mirror on
the wall . . .
stretch your
shoulder
nice and
tall.

Always keep your eyes on the weight you're lifting. This keeps you focused on what you're doing.

3. **Exhaling to a count of four, lower your right arm and turn your head forward to return to the starting position (see Figure 18-2a).**

   Don't slump your shoulders; keep them wide open so it feels as if your chest is smiling.

Repeat this exercise four to six times with each arm, pause to rest, and then do four to six more repetitions with each arm.

The Ticking Clock

Smooth, rhythmic movements are known to massage away stiffness in the body and aid in your ability to balance. The Ticking Clock gets its name because you move your body similarly to a clock pendulum. This exercise is about timed movement and the timeless quality of "being." It warms up the sides of your body and helps your neck and spine feel more flexible. It also stretches your shoulders and tones the muscles of your torso.

Grab your hand weights for this exercise and follow these steps:

1. **Sit in a chair with your arms hanging at your sides, the weights in your hands, and your palms facing inward (see Figure 18-3a).**

   This is the starting position. Look straight ahead.

2. **Turn your head to look over your right shoulder.**

   As you turn, keep your shoulders squared.

3. **As you exhale to a count of four, gently arc your torso to your right side (see Figure 18-3b).**

   Look down at the weight in your right hand, and feel your spine stretching.

4. **As you inhale to a count of four, return to the upright starting position (see Figure 18-3a).**

   Turn your head and look forward as you return to the starting position.

Alternating sides with each repetition, repeat this exercise four to six times on each side of your body, pause to rest, and then do four to six more repetitions on each side of your body.

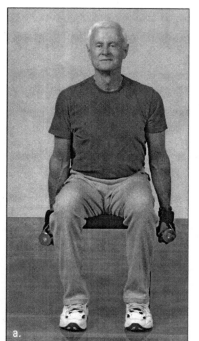 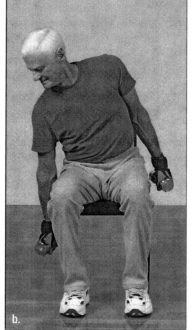

Figure 18-3:
Tick tock . . . tick tock . . . arc your body slowly in rhythm with your breathing.

a. b.

The Wave

Feeling a bit too tight and sore to surf the waves? Well, the yoga-with-weights wave is here to help. The Wave stretches your back and spine and releases tension from your head, neck, and shoulders. The rhythmic motion of the exercise also teaches you balance, coordination, and stability. For muscle benefit, the Wave strengthens and tones your abdominal muscles.

You need hand weights to do the yoga wave. When you're ready, follow these steps:

1. **Sit in a chair with your back separated from the back of the chair and your arms hanging down at your sides, holding the weights with your palms facing inward (see Figure 18-4a).**

   This is the starting position. Look straight ahead. If your back is touching the back of the chair, you may be tempted to rely on the chair for support, which would defeat the purpose of this exercise.

2. **Exhaling to a count of four, roll your shoulders up and over as you slowly lower the trunk of your body onto your thighs; let the weights hang beside your body as you lean forward (see Figure 18-4b).**

   Allow the weights to slowly pull you down. As you exhale, slowly push the air from your lungs so that by the time your body touches your thighs, you're pushing out the last bit of air.

   Anchor your buttocks to the chair to keep from slipping forward.

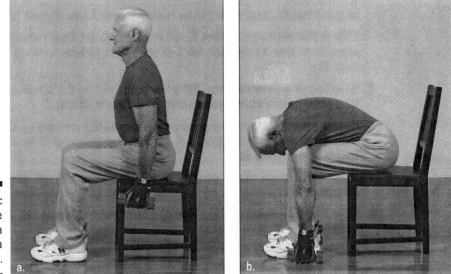

Figure 18-4: Move to the rhythm of a wave, not a tsunami.

Your head can hang down in this position. If you can't hang your head all the way, hang it as far as is comfortable, or lift your head slightly as you bend forward.

3. **Inhaling to a count of four, sit up and roll your shoulders up and back down again to return to the starting position (see Figure 18-4a).**

   Move your feet forward or backward if it helps you maintain your balance.

Repeat this exercise four to six times, pause to rest, and then do four to six more repetitions.

The Egyptian

If your declining range of motion is starting to make everyday tasks — like grabbing objects out of the cupboard — difficult to manage, you can fight back with exercises like the Egyptian. This exercise tones and strengthens your back, arms, chest, and shoulders. It also expands your chest and gives your shoulders a wider range of movement.

Draw your belly in and up throughout this exercise. Engaged belly muscles help you lift the weights and maintain stability.

To do the Egyptian, you need your hand weights. When you're ready, follow these steps:

1. **Sit in a chair with your arms hanging down to your sides, the weights in your hands, and your palms facing inward (see Figure 18-5a).**

   This is the starting position. Look straight ahead. Don't shrug your shoulders, lean against the back of the chair, or lean forward during this exercise.

2. **Inhaling to a count of four, lift your arms out to the sides until you join your hands above your head (see Figure 18-5b).**

   Rotate your hands so that your palms are facing upward by the time your arms are halfway lifted. Look up so that you're gazing at your hands above your head.

   If you can't reach above your head, lift your arms as high as you comfortably can.

3. **Exhaling to a count of four, slowly lower your arms to the starting position (see Figure 18-5a).**

   Rotate your hands again as you lower your arms so they end up facing inward at the starting position. Lower your gaze so that you're looking straight ahead as you lower your arms.

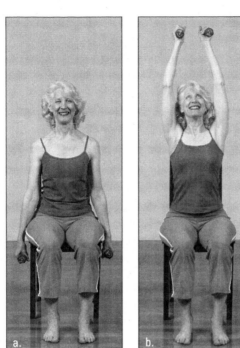

Figure 18-5:
The
Egyptian
improves
your posture
and your
range of
motion.

Repeat this exercise four to six times, pause to rest, and then do four to six more repetitions.

The Pigeon

The yoga-with-weights Pigeon isn't like those pigeons in the park that eat your picnic food and chirp away your peace and quite. This Pigeon increases the range of motion in your hips — if you're tight in this area, the Pigeon opens you up. The exercise also increases blood circulation to your hips and pelvic girdle, which helps you when you're climbing stairs or walking your dog.

Don't attempt this exercise without the permission of your primary caregiver if you've recently had a hip replacement.

Pick up both your hand weights and grab one ankle weight for this exercise. When you're ready, follow these steps:

1. **Sitting in a chair, place your right ankle over your left knee, and place the ankle weight on your right thigh.**

   The ankle weight helps anchor your thigh in place. By placing one leg over the other, you open and stretch out your hip and groin.

If you can't lift your ankle onto your knee, cross your ankles instead or put your foot on a footstool.

2. **Grab your hand weights, separate your arms as far apart as you can, and lift them to shoulder height with your elbows bent and palms facing forward (see Figure 18-6a).**

   This is the scarecrow position, and also your starting position. Make sure your spine is erect and that you're relaxed.

3. **Inhaling to a count of four, lift your arms overhead (see Figure 18-6b).**

   Lift to a place that's comfortable for you. In weightlifting terminology, this action is called an *overhead press* or *military press.*

4. **Exhaling to a count of four, lower the weights to the starting position (see Figure 18-6a).**

   Lower the weights slowly so you can feel your muscles working. Keep your belly muscles engaged for stability and balance.

Repeat this exercise four to six times with each leg, pause to rest, and then do four to six more repetitions with each leg.

Figure 18-6:
Look straight ahead, and look sharp, as you press your way to better mobility and circulation.

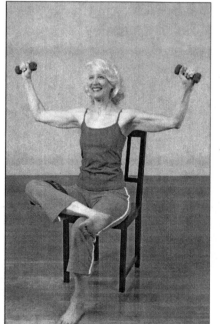
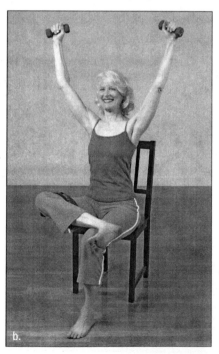

The Heart Lift

The Heart Lift is a great exercise for people of all ages, but it's especially helpful for seniors, because it brings a balance of oxygen and blood to your heart. The exercise opens and expands your chest and helps you to breathe more deeply. It also strengthens your spine, abdominal muscles, and quads. We call it the Heart Lift because the exercise brings you more joy and energy as it opens up your chest.

You need ankle weights for this exercise. When you're strapped up, follow these steps:

1. **Sit on the edge of a chair, and reach backward to grasp the back of the chair with your hands.**

   If you can't hold the back of the chair, hold the sides of the chair seat.

2. **Roll your shoulders up, back, and down; lift your chest; and raise your chin (see Figure 18-7a).**

   This is the starting position. Sink your buttocks deeply into the chair so you can lean forward slightly. Feel the front of your body stretching, and enjoy breathing in this position as your heart opens up.

3. **Exhaling to a count of four, lift your right knee a few inches and then straighten your right leg (see Figure 18-7b).**

   Press forward through your heel, and continue to hold on to the chair for balance.

4. **Inhaling to a count of four, lower your right leg to the starting position (see Figure 18-7a).**

   Lower your leg slowly to the rhythm of your breathing; don't drop it.

Figure 18-7:
Feel your heart open up as the oxygen enters and leaves your body.

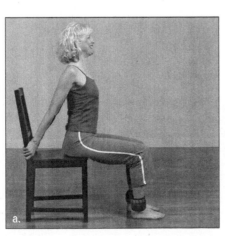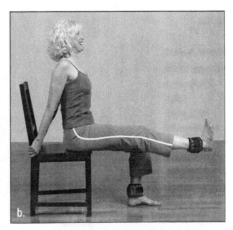

Alternating legs with each repetition, do this exercise four to six times with each leg, pause to rest, and then do four to six more repetitions with each leg.

The Hacker

The Hacker is a simple exercise that builds strength and flexibility in your lower body. The exercise works your quad and hamstring muscles while toning your belly and increasing the range of movement in your hips. The Hacker helps build the necessary strength for climbing up and down stairs and ladders.

Strap on your ankle weights for this exercise. Adding hand weights is an option for people who feel strong enough (the model in Figure 18-8 explores this option). When you're ready, follow these steps:

1. **Sit on a chair with your back separated from the back of the chair, your feet flat on the floor, and your arms hanging at your sides (see Figure 18-8a).**

   This is the starting position. Make sure your spine is erect and your shoulders are squared. If you want to use hand weights, hold them with your palms facing inward.

2. **Exhaling to a count of four, lift your right knee toward your chest (see Figure 18-8b).**

   Engage your belly muscles; you should feel these muscles working as you lift. Keep your foot flexed to engage your leg muscles.

Figure 18-8: Work your belly muscles and legs as you keep your trunk straight.

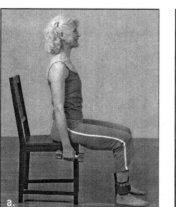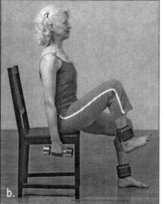

3. **Inhaling to a count of four, lower your leg to the starting position (see Figure 18-8a).**

   Lower your leg slowly; keep your leg muscles fully engaged all the way down.

Be careful not to lean forward as you do this exercise. Breathe deeply into your lower back.

Alternating legs with each repetition, do this exercise four to six times with each leg, pause to rest, and then do four to six more repetitions with each leg.

The Champion

The time has come for you to feel like a champion. The yoga-with-weights Champion strengthens, conditions, and tones the trunk of your body, your shoulders, and your arms; refines the integrity of your muscles; contributes to the structure of your bones; and brings more blood to your pelvic girdle, which helps with movement. You look like the champion of the world as you curl your arms (just don't wave to any imaginary crowd).

You need hand weights and ankle weights for this exercise. When you're ready, follow these steps:

1. **Straddle the right corner of a chair seat with your bent right knee in front of you over the chair, your left leg bent and at your side, and the toes of your left foot curled under for support.**

   Your left knee should be a couple of inches from the floor in this position. Make sure you have the hand weights in your hands at this point.

2. **Twist the trunk of your body slightly to the left, and lift and extend both of your arms to shoulder height, palms facing upward (see Figure 18-9a).**

   This is the starting position. Your shoulders should be directly above your hips. Look ahead toward the arm in front of you — your right arm in this case.

3. **Exhaling to a count of four, bend your elbows and lift the weights toward your shoulders (see Figure 18-9b).**

   In weightlifting terminology, this action is called a *bicep curl*.

4. **Inhaling to a count of four, extend your arms and return to the starting position (see Figure 18-9a).**

Repeat this exercise four to six times, pause to rest, and turn your body to the opposite side of the chair to do four to six more repetitions for the other side of your body.

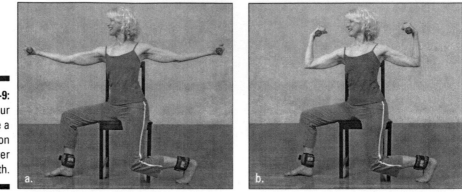

Figure 18-9:
Flex your
arms like a
champion
for better
health.

The Body Builder

The Body Builder exercises your buttocks and tones your legs, back, and thighs. This part of the workout builds the bone density in your back, spine, and legs, which allows you to feel free to be active without worrying about injury.

Wear ankle weights for this exercise. When you're strapped and ready to go, follow these steps:

1. **Standing behind a chair, hold the top of the chair with both hands and, bending at your waist, step backward far enough so that your trunk and arms are parallel to the floor (see Figure 18-10a).**

   This is the starting position.

   We suggest that you put the chair against a wall so that it doesn't slide when you do this exercise, which could cause you to slip and fall. (The model in Figure 18-10 didn't take our advice, but she's a daredevil.)

2. **Inhaling to a count of four, lift your right leg behind your body as high as you can without straining or causing too much discomfort (see Figure 18-10b).**

   Ideally, your leg should be parallel to the floor, but if you can't lift it that high, don't worry about it. You can bend your knee if you need to.

3. **Exhaling to a count of four, lower your leg to the starting position (see Figure 18-10a).**

   Lower your leg slowly and gently; don't drop it down.

Alternating legs with each repetition, do this exercise four to six times with each leg, pause to rest, and then do four to six more repetitions with each leg.

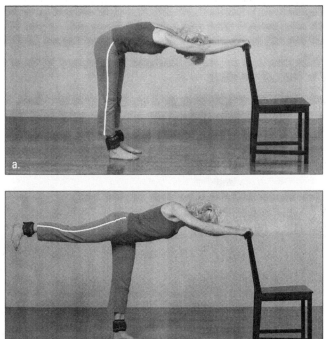

Figure 18-10:
Who says
body
builders
can't be
graceful
doing yoga?

The Triangle

The Triangle gives you the chance to really challenge your muscles and build strength. The exercise stretches the sides of your body and creates strength and stability in your arms, legs, and trunk.

You need both ankle weights and one hand weight for this exercise. When you're ready, follow these steps:

1. **Stand behind a chair with your legs apart, your right foot pointing to the chair, and your left foot at a 45-degree angle with respect to the chair.**

   Your body should be facing left when positioned behind the chair in this position. Your feet should be a little wider than your hips.

2. **Grasp the top of the chair with your left hand; with your right hand, hold the hand weight at your side, palm facing your body (see Figure 18-11a).**

   This is the starting position.

3. **Exhaling to a count of four, stretch the right side of your body by lifting the hand weight over and around your head. As you lift, turn your head to the left and bend your left elbow (see Figure 18-11b).**

    Press into your legs as you lift the hand weight, and try to arc the weight over the back of the chair.

    If you can't lift the weight over your body or over the chair, lift it as high as you comfortably can, or don't use the hand weight.

4. **Inhaling to a count of four, slowly return to the starting position (see Figure 18-11a).**

Repeat this exercise four to six times, pause to rest, and turn around to do four to six repetitions with the other side of your body.

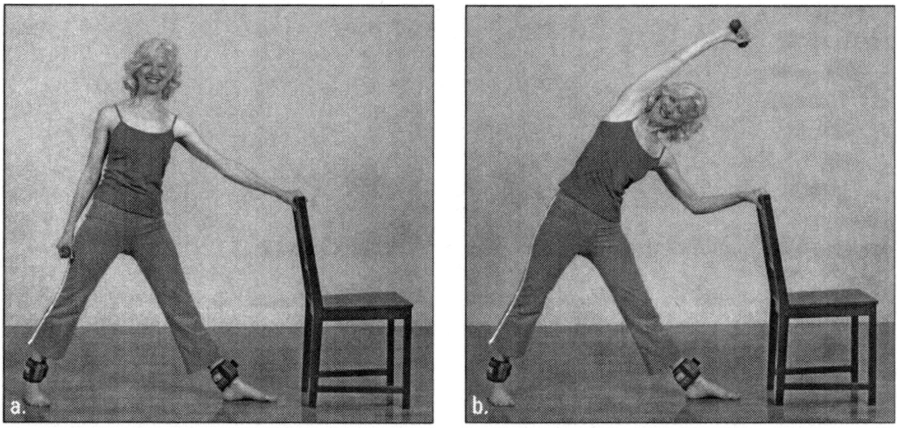

Figure 18-11:
Don't be a
square —
being a
triangle
strengthens
your body.

a. b.

The Lift

The Lift is a full-body exercise that lengthens the quad muscles in your legs and opens your groin. The exercise also tones and strengthens your spine and chest. As it tones your lower-body muscles, the Lift also exercises your arms — specifically your triceps.

You need both ankle weights and one hand weight for this exercise. When you're ready, follow these steps:

1. **Straddle the right corner of a chair seat with your bent right knee in front of you over the chair, your left leg bent and at your side, and the toes of your left foot curled under for support.**

   Your left knee should be close to the floor in this position. Make sure you're seated firmly in the chair with your right leg.

2. **Holding the hand weight with both hands, lift your hands above your head and bend your elbows so the weight goes behind your head (see Figure 18-12a).**

   This is the starting position. Your elbows should be near your ears; don't drop your head.

   If you can't reach your arms back far enough, reach them as far as you feel comfortable. You can also do this exercise without the hand weight.

3. **Inhaling to a count of four, straighten your arms and raise the weight over your head (see Figure 18-12b).**

4. **Exhaling to a count of four, lower the weight to the starting position (see Figure 18-12a).**

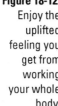

   Be careful not to hit yourself in the head on the way down.

Repeat this exercise four to six times, pause to rest, and then do four to six more repetitions.

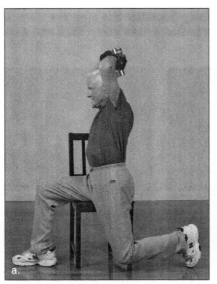 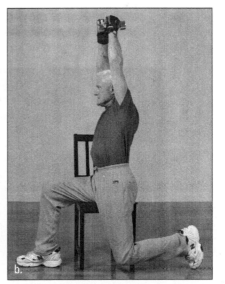

Figure 18-12: Enjoy the uplifted feeling you get from working your whole body.

The Seated Twist

The Seated Twist aims to wring your body out like a wet rag to make you feel more relaxed. The exercise loosens your neck and spine and releases tension from your shoulders and neck. It also increases the circulation in your legs, because when you cross and uncross your legs, you stimulate blood flow. Twisting and releasing your torso does the same.

Strap on your ankle weights and follow these steps:

1. **Sitting toward the front of a chair, cross your right leg over your left leg.**

   The weights on your ankles help anchor you into the chair.

2. **Place your left hand on the outside of your right knee, and reach your right hand behind you so you can hold the back of the chair at a location and level that's comfortable for you (see Figure 18-13a).**

   This is the starting position. Draw your belly in and up for support, and make sure that your spine is erect and your chin is slightly lifted.

3. **Exhaling to a count of four, turn your back, neck, and head one vertebrae at a time to look over your right shoulder (see Figure 18-13b).**

   Start your twist in the area behind your navel, and move upward in a spiraling direction. Imagine that your spine is twisting like a spiral staircase, with your mind climbing the stairs one step at a time. Twisting with an engaged abdomen protects your lower back and neck.

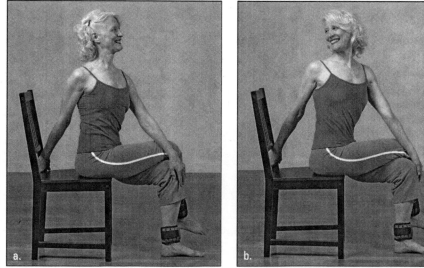

Figure 18-13:
Wring the tension from your body with the Seated Twist.

a.

b.

You can use your left hand, holding your crossed leg back, as leverage, which lengthens your spine and engages your core muscles even more.

4. **Inhaling to a count of four, rotate your back, neck, and head to the starting position (see Figure 18-13a).**

   Slowly unwind as you return to the starting position; don't jerk.

Repeat the exercise four to six times with this side of your body, pause to rest, and turn your body to the opposite side of the chair to do four to six more repetitions with the other side of your body.

Ending Meditation

Before you leave this workout, we encourage you to engage in meditation for a moment or two. Meditation requires mental focus and concentration, and in conjunction with the exercises we describe in this chapter, it helps unclutter your mind. Chapter 6 describes several meditation techniques. Find a technique that you enjoy and do it before you move on with your day.

Part V
Addressing Special Situations

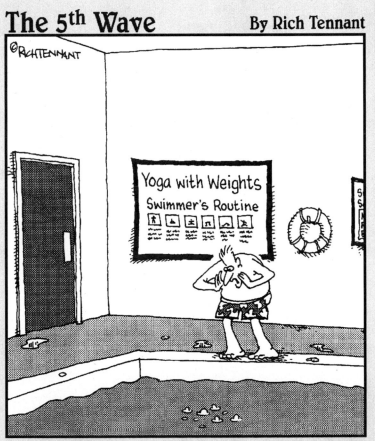

The 5th Wave   By Rich Tennant

Yoga with Weights
Swimmer's Routine

"I know it's a swimmer's routine, but I'm pretty sure it's supposed to be performed outside the pool."

In this part . . .

The other parts of this book show you how yoga with weights benefits everybody. Part V shows you how yoga with weights can benefit three select groups: athletes, seniors, and women.

Whether you hit the courts on the weekends or spend your weekdays as an all-pro MVP, we show you how yoga-with-weights exercises can help you perform better in the sport you love most. We also look at women's health issues and demonstrate how yoga with weights can benefit pregnant women. Finally, we include gentle yoga-with-weights exercises designed especially for seniors.

Chapter 19

Ten Ways to Stay Motivated

The hardest part of any workout is taking the first step, lifting the first weight, or taking the first deep breath. Getting motivated is harder than bench-pressing, harder than running through the park, and harder than any yoga-with-weights exercise. When you're motivated to exercise, working out comes easy, but when you don't feel motivated, starting your workout can seem like pushing a boulder up a hillside.

This chapter gives you ten ways to get yourself motivated. When you can't seem to find the time, when you're overcome by listlessness, or when you're dead tired, turn to this chapter.

A little bit each day makes a big difference! You can do as little as two or three 30-minute yoga-with-weights workouts each week and see a significant improvement in your health and mental state. Make the commitment, and you'll feel a surge of energy and tremendous pride in what you're accomplishing.

Take a Deep Breath

When you suddenly feel a lack of motivation, try taking a deep breath. Whether you're getting up your gumption to start a yoga-with-weights workout, to mow the yard, or to wash the dishes, stop for a moment to pay attention to your breathing. Take a deep, slow, gentle breath, and feel the air filling your lungs. Relax as you feel the air exiting your lungs. Doing this helps you take stock of yourself and build up the motivation to get started. Three to ten deep breaths can shift the cycle of your energy and the direction of your thinking.

Consciously breathing helps you stay more alert and focus on the present, not on day-to-day worries, past regrets, or current responsibilities. It helps you notice what you're feeling at the present moment — without judgment. And it gives you clarity so you can confront the task at hand, whatever it may be.

Breathing is an important — some would say essential — part of traditional yoga and yoga-with-weights practices. We devote Chapter 4 to breathing, in case you don't know the proper way to breathe or if you want to discover many different ways to breathe.

Make the Commitment to Exercise

One way to make the commitment to exercise is to make it at night before you go to sleep. Before you hit the pillow, set your alarm clock an hour earlier than usual, place it across the room so that you have to get out of bed to turn it off, and put your walking shoes and the workout clothes that you like to wear next to it. Instead of lying in bed after your alarm clock goes off and hitting the snooze button, you have to get out of bed to turn the alarm off. And because you're out of bed, you may as well put on your exercise clothes and shoes. You can start walking or running outside or on a treadmill right away. (Chapter 6 lists the benefits of walking before a yoga-with-weights workout or just for the sake of walking.)

When you're finished warming up, choose which yoga-with-weights workout you want to do, and get to it. Which workout you do depends on your physical, mental, and emotional needs. Every day is different, and you have plenty of workouts to choose from in this book. You can finish most of the workouts in 20 to 30 minutes.

Here's another tactic to use: When you wake up in the morning, make a mental or, better yet, written list of the things you want to accomplish during the day, and include a yoga-with-weights workout on your list. Writing goals down in list form helps you accomplish important tasks.

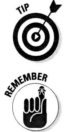

Three and four o'clock in the afternoon are good times to do a yoga-with-weights workout, if you can find the time. Most people have a snack in the afternoon to get their energy to complete the day, but a yoga-with-weights workout is more energizing than a snack, and it's healthier, too. You get the strength for that last uphill push before dinnertime, and you feel good about yourself because you completed your daily yoga-with-weights workout.

Take Care of Yourself

Taking care of your body makes you healthier and happier, which enables you to give more of yourself to any task you want to accomplish and to other people in your life. In the course of a day, life makes all kinds of demands on you. Your job, your spouse, and your children all require you to be certain places and do certain things. It may seem selfish for you to set aside these responsibilities for a moment to focus on you, but taking care of yourself actually has benefits for the people you love and the people who depend on you. Nourishing yourself gives you the power and strength to nourish others. Instead of feeling exhausted and tired (and maybe resentful as a result), you can be a light to other people. The more you take care of yourself, the more you have to offer others.

Celebrate the Benefits to Your Sex Life

As advertisers know, sex is a powerful motivator. Why else do so many models appear in advertisements? You can use sex to motivate you to do your yoga-with-weights exercises, because yoga with weights can improve your sex life. The exercises in this book boost your metabolism and increase your ability to focus and concentrate. You'll feel healthier and better, and you'll notice improvements in your self-esteem and stamina. All these benefits have the effect of making you more confident and alive in the bedroom.

Another benefit to your sex life comes from the emphasis that yoga with weights places on breathing. Many sexual techniques call on you to focus on your breathing as a means of relaxing and enhancing the sensation so you enjoy sex more. Relaxation occurs naturally in the breathing practices as the body releases stress and the habitually thinking mind quiets down. You become more receptive, present, and relaxed when you can focus on and control your breathing. Relaxation is supportive to sexual arousal and enhanced duration. You feel increased energy and pleasure, and you can begin to experience the timeless quality of sexual fulfillment.

The exercises in this book show you how to control your breathing to relax and to focus your energy. We give breathing an entire chapter in this book — Chapter 4. We don't mind, and we won't tattletale, if you use the breathing techniques in this book in the bedroom as well as the gym.

322 Part VI: The Part of Tens

Reward Yourself

Go ahead and reward yourself with a piece of chocolate when you complete a yoga-with-weights workout. You deserve a reward, especially if the prospect of getting a reward motivates you to exercise.

You'll discover after you do several workouts, however, that the exercises are rewards in and of themselves. After a 20-minute workout, you feel refreshed; you feel like you've caught your second wind; and you feel alive, inspired, and ready to take on the rest of your day.

Consider How Well You're Sleeping

According to the National Sleep Foundation (www.sleepfoundation.org), fewer than half of all Americans sleep long enough or well enough. Sleep deprivation depresses your immune system, increases irritability, and slows your reaction time. Losing sleep can also accelerate the aging process.

All forms of exercise help you sleep better, because exercise is the best anti-dote for stress, and stress is what usually causes sleeplessness. Yoga with weights may be the best answer to your sleep problems, because the exercise program helps you relax and de-stress.

If you're the kind of person who gets revved up on account of stress, exercising uses up your excess energy so you can sleep. If you're the type of person who feels overwhelmed and listless as a result of stress, exercising helps you achieve clarity so you feel less overwhelmed and more tired. Exercise helps regulate and balance your ability to sleep naturally.

 If you wake up agitated in the middle of the night, or if you're suffering from insomnia, try taking the long, slow, yogic breaths we describe in Chapter 4. Or try this technique: Lie on your bed with your eyes closed and your hands resting on your belly. As you inhale, feel your belly expand and rise to the ceiling. As you exhale, feel it softly contract, and visualize your belly drawing closer to your spine. By focusing on the rise and fall of your belly as you breathe, you still and soothe your mind. You quiet your thoughts and, in doing so, permit yourself to fall asleep. Deep-belly breathing helps trigger the relaxation response in your brain.

Set Your Sights on a Goal

You want to look good at your high-school reunion, don't you? Many people don't attend their reunions because they don't feel good about their lives and their appearances. Yoga with weights empowers your body, mind, and spirit. Six-month's worth of yoga-with-weights exercises will have you looking good and sporting a greater sense of joy and confidence to reconnect with friends from your past. Don't be surprised if your former classmates marvel at how youthful you are and how little you've changed from your yearbook photo. When your classmates ask, "How did you do it?" and "What's your secret?" you can tell them about your yoga-with-weights exercise regimen, or you can give them a wink, shrug your shoulders, and act mysterious. It's up to you.

Find a Workout Partner

Working out with a friend turns exercising into a social occasion. It makes exercising more fun, and you and your friend can encourage one another to try harder and to exercise regularly. Your friend can also be your teacher. He or she can tell you when you aren't lifting your leg high enough or stretching your arm far enough. (Chapter 3 gives you tips on working out in a group setting.)

A little healthy competition between workout partners is a good thing. As your partner encourages you, you'll want to try harder. Working with a partner also gives you the opportunity to be a teacher. You get to practice being kind and encouraging when you see he or she having a hard time.

Talk to Yourself

Before you start a workout, talk yourself into it. Tell yourself about all the health benefits you'll enjoy after your yoga-with-weights workout. And give yourself a pep talk in the middle of a workout when you start to wilt. Tell yourself that you have only a few more exercises to go, and remind yourself that it's only a matter of minutes before you catch your second wind. Think about how good you'll feel when you finish. Recall the feeling of pride and satisfaction you always get from a good workout.

Sometimes in the middle of a workout, a demon perches on your shoulder and tells you how tired you are and how easy it would be to quit right now. Put aside this kind of unhealthy self-talk. Shake off the demon and forge ahead.

Create a Workout Routine You Enjoy

After you do several different workouts from this book, you'll find a dozen or so exercises that you like most. Combine these exercises into a workout you enjoy. You don't have to work as hard to motivate yourself to do this self-made workout because it has your favorite exercises, which means you'll do it more often.

Chapter 15 explains how you can fashion your personal yoga-with-weights workout.

Chapter 20

Ten Myths about Yoga with Weights

Some people hear the word "yoga" and think of swamis or men in loincloths meditating on mountaintops. We respectfully suggest that modern-day yoga is quite different from this image. Yoga, like yoga practitioners, is flexible, which explains why it can branch off into separate but related disciplines such as yoga with weights. The discipline has one foot in modern times and one foot in ancient India. But because yoga originates in India, a foreign and exotic land, a few myths have evolved around the practice. This chapter aims to dispel these myths and show how yoga has been transformed over the years into a new discipline.

You Must Be Flexible

It's easy to see why some people believe you must be a contortionist to study yoga or yoga with weights. Books and magazine articles about yoga invariably show photographs of people twisting themselves into pretzel-like positions and poses.

After looking at the photographs, some people conclude that you must be flexible, and we mean really flexible, to practice yoga. People who can't touch their toes or have trouble widening their shoulders may conclude that yoga with weights isn't for them.

Most of the people you see in the photographs, however, have been studying yoga for years. When they started their yoga adventures, they may not have been able to touch their toes. As you'll discover after you do yoga-with-weights exercises for a few weeks, flexibility isn't necessarily something you're born with. Even if you're stiff as a board, you can become flexible with persistence and practice. In our yoga classes, we've seen students who could hardly bend over without creaking like a rusty gate turn into graceful, flexible yoga practitioners. It happens all the time. With a little practice, the caterpillar can turn into a butterfly.

If you're not flexible, you're an ideal candidate for yoga with weights. Start slowly, never force your body, and work at your own level of ability. Be consistent, and you'll see change. Improving your flexibility also improves your circulation, straightens your posture, makes you stronger, lowers the risk of muscle strains, decreases your risk of bodily injury, and, most important of all, enlarges your capacity to enjoy life. Yoga helps you gain flexibility not only in your body, but also in your mind and heart.

You Can't Balance While Holding Weights

Balance is an essential part of the yoga-with-weights discipline. Balancing teaches you to focus and concentrate, helps align the muscles of your body, and improves your posture. People who have had yoga lessons or are familiar with yoga see the weights and may say to themselves, "That's not yoga. How can you balance with weights in your hands and weights on your ankles?"

However, we believe that carrying a small amount of additional weight actually brings more balance to the yoga discipline. The extra challenge of bearing the weight makes you stronger and challenges your ability to concentrate even more. You have to pull deeper into the core muscles of your trunk and torso as you balance, which makes your core muscles stronger.

Yoga-with-weights exercises require you to hold 1- to 5-pound weights in your hands or strap them on your ankles (you can choose which amount of weight you want in each exercise). You'll be surprised to discover how much intensity, improved focus, and balance this small amount of weight brings to the yoga discipline.

Yoga Is a Religion

Yoga comes from the Sanskrit word *yuj*, which means "to join" or "to unite." The yoga practitioner should unite the body and the mind to achieve self-realization. In India and in some yoga studios in the West, yoga practitioners burn incense, display statues of deities, and chant. All this can make yoga sound and feel like a religion, but in reality, the Indian trappings are part of the mystique, spirituality, and charm of India expressing itself freely in yoga studios. They aren't religious manifestations. The bottom line is that yoga comes from a rich and varied spiritual tradition. Connecting with that tradition brings a certain depth to your study of yoga with weights. Can you practice yoga without all the trappings? Absolutely. And we're here to prove it with the yoga-with-weights workout.

The yoga practice does offer a system of philosophy to support mental clarity and awareness, emotional balance, and physical well-being. Yoga is the oldest known system of self-development. It carries the philosophy of "anything is possible." The real beauty of yoga is that it supports your everyday living in practical and real ways. Yoga isn't a religion; it's a spiritual lifestyle. Depending on what you want to make of it and how deeply you want to explore the ancient discipline and practices, yoga is more of an exploration of self, a journey of discovery, and a path to enhance your awareness and connection to life.

In the beginning, most people come to yoga with weights to improve their health or to try out a novel form of exercise. Over time, some casual practitioners discover the spiritual aspects along with the physical benefits of yoga. The physical benefits speak for themselves. As your body thrives in the yoga practice, your mind clears. Life becomes an opportunity to grow and develop yourself. Yoga with weights can quiet your mind and help you get in touch with yourself and your surroundings. It can give you spiritual clarity, but the discipline doesn't take away from any faith or religion that you believe in; it only empowers you to be discerning and to find out what's best for you. Practicing yoga doesn't keep you from practicing the religion of your choice; it enhances all the things you're interested in and gives you more energy to enjoy these things.

You Must Be a Vegetarian

Yoga originated in India, and for that reason it carries with it many associations with that nation, one being vegetarianism and the principal of not harming any living being. Still, you can practice yoga with weights without being a vegetarian. Vegetarianism and the choice of foods you eat are personal choices. Some of the greatest yoga teachers are vegetarians; other great teachers eat meat. You can practice the yoga-with-weights system without adopting any of the customs or beliefs that are associated with yoga.

Traditional yoga emphasizes that your body is wise and that you should listen to your body. Yoga is a system of self-knowledge, so it's up to you to explore and balance your body's health with the right foods that work for you. Use the tips and suggestions we provide in Chapter 13 to improve your diet. If you feel that you need the protein from meat for energy, feel free to eat meat. And if you decide that the cleansing benefits you get from eliminating meat from your diet are necessary for your health, you can stop eating meat and adopt a vegetarian diet. The choice is always yours.

Yoga with Weights Is for Super-Trendy Health Freaks

Some of the people who practice yoga are super-trendy health freaks. You know the type: the tall, toned, lean, slender, buff body; the trendy clothes made with hemp or fabrics imported from India; and the intricate tattoo running down the spine.

Yoga has become a multi-billion-dollar industry in the past decade. Celebrities such as Madonna practice yoga. You can see fashionable people in loose-fitting "yoga wear" on the streets of Beverly Hills and other chi-chi locales.

We hope that these trendy trappings don't prevent anyone from trying yoga with weights. Yoga is at least 5,000 years old, it defies fashion trends, and it has permanent appeal. Don't be afraid to try it because you're not a super-trendy health freak.

Yoga Makes You Wimpy

Yoga has a reputation for being a passive form of exercise, even if you add weights. It isn't a competitive sport (although it helps you to identify your issues with competition and how these issues may be getting in the way of real success; see Chapter 16 for more on yoga with weights and sports). Yoga practitioners don't get pumped-up angry or roar at their opponents, because they don't have opponents. Furthermore, the idea behind yoga with weights is to build strength from within, not to build strength by struggling with an opponent or a piece of exercise equipment.

On the other hand, yoga isn't really a passive form of exercise. It organizes your strength, internal energy, and awareness. Yoga builds strength in areas that other exercise programs don't come near. It builds self-confidence, quiets your mind, and helps you find your own direction. You develop your inner as well as your outer strength. Does that sound wimpy to you? Kareem Abdul-Jabbar, John McEnroe, and Dan Marino don't think so. These professional athletes practiced yoga in their playing days and continue to practice it now.

You Have to Be Very Coordinated

You've probably seen photographs of a yogi standing on one leg, with his other leg tucked into his groin and his hands spread wide. Many yoga-with-weights exercises require you to balance this way, and seeing the photographs may lead you to believe that you have to be very coordinated to do yoga-with-weights exercises.

We're happy to report that balancing, like flexibility, is an acquired skill. Day by day, exercise by exercise, you get better at balancing. You don't have to be coordinated to begin with, because the exercises teach you to be coordinated. Many students have come into our classes unable, for example, to turn their bodies without leading with their eyes. This is a sure sign that these students have been coursing their way through life with levels of unconscious movement that challenge their bodies to try to keep up with their eyes. This can be exhausting, cause chronic discomfort, wear out the body before its time, and cause mental exhaustion. The balancing exercises we instruct have taught these students how to trust their bodies and move themselves with self-assurance and poise.

Balance is one of the overlooked benefits of the yoga-with-weights exercise regimen. The balancing exercises teach you how to use different muscles in consort — how to flex some muscles and relax others. The purpose of balancing exercises is to help you explore your sensory pathways and the muscles of your body while strengthening both. Balancing is an important part of the yoga-with-weights goal of making you more self-aware of and confident in your body.

You Have to Go Away to Do It

You can find beautiful descriptions of yoga retreats all over the Internet. In fact, we occasionally lead yoga retreats to exotic places (see the appendix for some listings). As wonderful as these yoga retreats are, they've led some people to the erroneous idea that you can only do yoga exercises at retreats or spas, or that you have to go away to create the right environment to practice yoga.

You can do your yoga-with-weights workout anyplace in the world where you can find a few square feet of exercise space. Except for thumb twiddling, which requires even less exercise space, yoga is the most mobile of all exercise programs. You can do it in a hotel room, on the beach, or in a tree house. All you need is the will to start exercising and a few square feet of flat ground or floor space. (See Chapter 3 for tips on creating your own workout space.)

You Must Have a Certain Body Type

You don't have to be slim or slender to do a yoga-with-weights workout. In fact, many traditional yogis are on the rotund side and look as if they don't work out regularly. Yoga practitioners come in all shapes, sizes, and ages. As far as appearance, the only thing yoga practitioners have in common is a healthy glow of fitness.

You Must Be Fit and Young

The myth that you have to be young and fit to practice yoga arose because people who do yoga look young and fit — especially people who do yoga with weights. For some people, doing yoga-with-weights exercises can be like drinking from the fountain of youth. They make you feel younger and great and keep you looking your best.

No age limit prohibits you from starting to study yoga with weights. If you don't believe us, check out Chapter 18, which shows photos of senior citizens doing the exercises. Yoga with weights can benefit people of all ages. As yoga instructors, we've been inspired many times over by our older students, who have the vibrancy and vitality of people half their age.

Chapter 21

Ten Ways to Chart Your Progress

In This Chapter

▶ Monitoring your appearance and weight

▶ Noticing your newfound mental alertness

▶ Tracking your strength and stamina

*H*ow can you tell if you're making progress in your yoga-with-weights exercise program? You can consult a tarot-card reader, or you can try the ten techniques we describe in this chapter.

Charting your progress when you undertake a new exercise program is more important than most people realize. In order to stick with it and know that you're doing it right, you need to be able to read the signs. This chapter helps you do just that by describing benchmarks of progress for yoga-with-weights practitioners.

Monitor Your Weight

If your yoga-with-weights goal is to lose weight, one of the surest ways to tell if an exercise program is helping you meet your goal is to weigh yourself. If you're shedding pounds, take it as a sign that you're exercising regularly and exercising well.

When tracking your weight, weigh yourself once a week at most, or perhaps once every two weeks or even once a month. Don't be obsessive about it. The problem with weighing yourself daily is that your body has natural weight fluctuations. For example, most people gain weight on the weekend, when they eat and rest more, so they weigh more on Monday morning than on Friday morning. You may also gain weight when you're on vacation, a time when you eat differently. You may also be retaining water. If you weigh yourself during a fluctuation and discover that you've gained weight, you may become needlessly discouraged.

Another factor to consider when you weigh yourself is that muscle weighs more than fat. You're replacing the fat you're burning with muscle, and you aren't losing weight for that reason in spite of exercising. Don't be discouraged; be proud of your stronger body.

 You lose weight when you exercise because you burn calories, but also for another important reason: Exercising increases your body temperature, which suppresses your appetite. When you feel the urge for a mid-afternoon snack, do a yoga-with-weights workout first, and make sure you consume plenty of water during the day. You'll burn calories, suppress your desire to eat, and eat a smaller snack.

Keep Tabs on Your Physical Energy

A sure-fire way to chart your progress is to gauge your physical energy. You'll feel more energized if you consistently do yoga-with-weights workouts. But how can you tell if you have more energy? You'll know if you have the energy to do the activities you want to do in your daily life. Walking uphill is easier. Housework isn't so much drudgery. In general, you feel more joyful, happy, and creative.

Look in the Mirror

One of these days an inventor will come up with a mirror that flatters and wheedles. And said inventor will become a millionaire. Until the flattering mirror arrives, however, gazing at yourself in a mirror is one of the best ways to tell if you're progressing in your exercise program.

Look at your complexion. Do you have a healthy glow? Is your skin shiny? Do your eyes sparkle? These signs tell you that you're progressing with your yoga-with-weights exercise regimen.

Check Your Clothes for Comfort

Isn't it a great feeling when you put on a pair of pants that used to cramp your waist but now feel loose? How comfortable your clothes are is another way to mark your exercise progress. When you feel better in your clothes, and when you don't have to hold your breath to get into your pants anymore, take it as a sign that you've lost weight and that your exercise program is working for you.

Your waistline seems to be the measuring stick for determining whether you fit into your clothes or have to squeeze into them, but how tight your clothes are around your hips, buttocks, and thighs also tells you if your clothes fit. Look at it this way: If you lose enough weight, you'll need a new wardrobe. Think of all the fun you can have shopping for new clothes.

Try keeping a pair of pants, a shirt, or a dress with which to measure your success. For example, put aside a pair of pants when you start exercising, and from time to time, as you lose weight, try on the pants and notice how slim you're getting.

Take Notice of What People Say

"You look great!" When someone gives you a compliment, you want to purr like a cat. And these kinds of compliments encourage you to stick to your regimen. You can chart your progress by the number of compliments you get.

Observe Your Mental Alertness

Most people associate being in shape with being physically fit, but being in shape also means that you're more alert mentally. Television quiz-show answers leap into your head, whereas before you had the "I have it on the tip of my tongue" feeling. Mentally, you don't have to work as hard. The answers come easier to you.

After a workout or after your walking warm-up (see Chapter 6), test how mentally alert you are. Compare your state of mental alertness on days when you work out to days when you don't work out. Can you stay on task? Does your work come easier? Are you more creative? You'll notice a real difference after you practice yoga with weights.

Use a Training Diary

A training diary helps you track your exercise progress. If you put a mark on your calendar whenever you finish a yoga-with-weights workout, you know right away how often you work out.

Sherri has a client who keeps a calendar in the room where she works out. This client proudly shows Sherri each week how many times she's worked out and what kinds of workouts she has done. Her diary gives her a real sense of accomplishment.

Training diaries have now entered the digital age. You can download training diaries from the Internet. Online diaries allow you to track the different exercises you do in a workout and generate graphs and charts that show how often and how intensively you work out. Some of the digital training diaries even work on hand-held computers.

Go to Cnet.com (www.cnet.com) to read about digital training diaries and to download trial versions of the programs (enter Training Diaries in the search box). The following are the leading digital diaries:

- ✔ **The Athlete's Diary:** Keep track of your fitness activities. (www.stevenscreek.com)
- ✔ **BYOB-Lite:** BYOB stands for "build your own body," not "bring your own bottle." (www.lexabean.com)
- ✔ **Exercise Diary:** A "fitness-tracking" software. (www.silveronion.com)

Recognize Your Feelings of Gratitude and Peace of Mind

Feeling bad, we believe, can be a habitual pattern and, in some cases, an addiction. You become so used to thinking negatively that you can't stop doing it, even if you know the consequences. You need to break these negative-thinking cycles and establish a new way of thinking.

Six weeks of eating right and exercising regularly seems to be the norm for breaking negative thought patterns. Doing yoga-with-weights exercises can really help you in this regard. The exercises create an internal shift; you can step back from your thoughts and notice the same thought patterns appearing again and again. The exercises help you let go of negativity and change how you feel physically and mentally. You'll feel better about yourself, and you won't sweat the little things.

Yoga-with-weights techniques will help to bring about a deeper connection to the self and provide a way of helping you to pay attention to your thoughts. Gratitude needs to be cultivated and encouraged. Be patient and give it time.

Reap the Benefits of Proper Breathing

Most people don't breathe properly. They take shallow breaths, or they tend to hold their breath. Yoga with weights — by strengthening your chest and lungs and making you conscious of how you breathe — can show you how to breathe in such a way that you relax and get the proper amount of oxygen. (Chapter 4 looks into breathing in detail.)

If you stick with yoga with weights long enough, the moment will come when you understand just how valuable breathing properly is. Perhaps you'll come to a stoplight in traffic, and instead of sighing, you'll take a yogic breath. You'll feel relaxation flooding your body, and you'll be fully present like no time before. You'll start noticing the details in the world around you — and the world will look pretty nice.

Most people who study yoga have a mini-epiphany. When you discover the value of proper breathing, consider it a benchmark moment. You'll know you're making great progress in your yoga-with-weights exercise program.

Feel Your Increased Endurance and Stamina

If you stick with your yoga-with-weights workout, you'll acquire more endurance and stamina. One of the features of these exercises is that they help you focus and concentrate, and in so doing, they help you develop endurance and stamina. You can stay with an activity longer because you have the strength of mind to focus for longer periods of time.

Because of your newfound stamina, you start saying "yes" to activities to which you previously said "no." The backpacking trip, the Proust novel, the extra project at work — you say "yes" to these activities because you know you can complete them and because you're willing to try more activities. You feel safe and confident in your own body, and you know your body will support you.

Appendix

Resources

• •

*T*his appendix lists resources for yoga-with-weights practitioners. You'll find Web sites; stores where you can buy equipment; magazines, books, and videos; spas and retreats; and organizations that specialize in yoga. As yet, yoga with weights is a young yoga discipline, so finding resources isn't easy; however, as the discipline grows, many of the resources we list are sure to jump on the bandwagon. Jump aboard while you still have room!

Yoga-with-Weights Web Sites

The following Web sites deal with yoga with weights:

- **Baptiste Power of Yoga:** Sherri Baptiste's yoga Web site. www.power ofyoga.com
- **Yoga with Weights:** Sherri Baptiste's Web site devoted to yoga with weights. www.yogawithweights.com

Yoga Mats and Clothing

You can often buy yoga mats and clothing at sporting goods stores and yoga centers; otherwise, you can look to the following online stores and companies for quality yoga mats and yoga clothing:

- **Hugger Mugger Yoga Products:** www.huggermugger.com
- **Marika:** www.marika.com
- **Prana:** www.prana.com
- **Shakti Shanti Yoga Wear:** www.shaktishantiyogawear.com
- **Vermont Soap — Yoga Mat Wash:** www.vermontsoap.com
- **Yoga Site:** www.yogasite.com

Hand and Ankle Weights

You can buy hand and ankle weights at sporting goods stores. The following reputable online stores also offer hand weights and ankle weights you can use for your yoga-with-weights workouts:

- **Heavyhands Hand Weights:** www.heavyhandsfitness.com
- **Mega Fitness:** megafitness.com/index.html
- **Nefitco.com:** www.nefitco.com/ankle.html
- **Perform Better:** www.performbetter.com
- **Theraband Soft Small Hand-Held Weights:** www.fitter1.com/theraband-soft-weights.html
- **Weider:** www.weiderfitness.com

Yoga and Health Magazines

Here are some yoga and health magazines worth investigating:

- *Alternative:* Provides the latest information about alternative and complementary health therapies. www.alternativemedicine.com
- *FIT* and *Fit Yoga:* Provide articles on yoga and fitness. www.fitmag.com
- *Healing Lifestyles & Spas:* Besides the excellent articles, you can find a spa in your area from this magazine's Web site. www.healinglifestyles.com
- *Men's & Women's Health:* This magazine provides tips and articles on fitness, nutrition, relationships, sex, careers, and lifestyle choices. www.menshealth.com and www.womenshealthmag.com
- *O:* Oprah Winfrey's magazine offers tips on health and exercise. www.oprah.com
- *Oxygen:* This magazine is devoted to women's fitness. www.getbig.com/magazine/oxygen/oxygen.htm
- *Prevention:* Offers advice for living a healthier life. www.prevention.com
- *Strength and Health:* A magazine for weightlifters. www.yorkbarbell.com/sandh.html

- ✔ *Yoga International:* Offers articles and insight into the yoga practice. www.yimag.org
- ✔ *Yoga Journal:* Web site of the longest-running yoga magazine. www.yogajournal.com

Books about Yoga, Fitness, and Diet

We recommend the following books about yoga, fitness, and diet:

- ✔ *Anatomy of Hatha Yoga,* by Timothy McCall, MD (Body and Breath, Inc.)
- ✔ *Forty Days to Personal Revolution,* by Baron Baptiste (Simon and Schuster)
- ✔ *Iron Yoga,* by Anthony Carillo (Rodale Books)
- ✔ *Journey into Power,* by Baron Baptiste (Simon and Schuster)
- ✔ *Meditation For Dummies,* by Stephan Bodian and Dean Ornish (Wiley)
- ✔ *Mind-Body Fitness For Dummies,* by Therese Iknoian (Wiley)
- ✔ *The New Detox Diet: The Complete Guide for Lifelong Vitality with Recipes, Menus, and Detox Plans,* by Elson Haas, MD, and Daniella Chace (Celestial Arts)
- ✔ *Nutrition For Dummies, 3rd Edition,* by Carol Ann Rinzler (Wiley)
- ✔ *Staying Healthy with Nutrition,* by Elson M. Haas (Celestial Arts)
- ✔ *Stop Your Cravings,* by Jennifer Workman (Free Press)
- ✔ *Strength Training Anatomy,* by Fredric Delavier (Human Kinetics Publishers)
- ✔ *Vitamins For Dummies,* by Christopher Hobbs and Elson Haas (Wiley)
- ✔ *Weight Training For Dummies,* by Liz Neporent and Suzanne Schlosberg (Wiley)
- ✔ *Woman's Book of Yoga and Health,* by Linda Sparrowe and Patricia Walden (Shambhala Publications)
- ✔ *Yoga For Dummies,* by Georg Feuerstein, Larry Payne, and Lilias Folan (Wiley)
- ✔ *Yoga RX,* by Larry Payne, Richard Usatine, Merry Aronson, and Rachelle Gardner (Broadway)

Videos about Yoga

Here are some video sources of information about yoga:

- **Power of Yoga:** Click the Music/Video link. www.powerofyoga.com
- **Samata Yoga:** Offers yoga books as well as videos. www.samata.com
- **Yoga with Weights:** Offers videos about yoga with weights and information about yoga-with-weights resources. www.yogawithweights.com
- **Yoga.com:** Offers videos about yoga (as well as books, clothing, and mats). www.yoga.com

Directories and Web Sites for Yoga, Health, and Fitness

You can search for a yoga class at these Web sites:

- **Mind Body Medical Institute:** Massachusetts-based nonprofit educational organization devoted to the study of the mind-body connection — especially the relaxation response. www.mbmi.org
- **Yoga Directory:** Search for yoga centers, classes, and studios. www.yoga-centers-directory.net
- **Yoga Finder:** Find yoga classes in your area. www.yogafinder.com
- **Yoga Journal:** This online yoga magazine offers a directory of yoga teachers (click the Class Search link). www.yogajournal.com

Yoga Retreats and Spas

The following yoga retreats and spas offer getaways where you can concentrate solely on your yoga practice:

- **Baptiste Bootcamps:** Intense yoga retreats and instruction from Baron Baptiste. www.baronbaptiste.com
- **Canyon Ranch:** A yoga retreat in the Berkshires. www.canyonranch.com
- **Golden Door:** A yoga retreat in Escondido, California. www.goldendoor.com
- **Kripalu Center for Yoga and Health:** A yoga retreat in beautiful Lenox, Massachusetts. www.kripalu.org

- **Power of Yoga Meditation Retreats:** Retreats are held at yoga and Zen retreat centers; beginners are welcome. www.powerofyoga.com

- **Rancho La Puerta:** A yoga retreat in Tecate, Baja California, Mexico. www.rancholapuerta.com

- **Spas Finder:** Click the Find Spas link to find a spa in your area. www.spafinder.com

- **Spa Spirit:** Personalized health and yoga retreats by Michele Hébert, a distinguished yoga teacher trained by Walt Baptiste. www.spaspirit.com

Fitness Centers That Offer Yoga Classes

Besides your local gyms and fitness centers, you can find yoga classes at the following gym franchises:

- **Gold's Gym's:** Gold's has over 550 health clubs nationwide. www.goldsgym.com

- **Nautilus:** Nautilus gyms are located in California. www.nautilusofmarin.com

- **Western Athletic/Bay Clubs:** You can find these clubs in Washington and California. www.westernathleticclubs.com

Yoga Study Centers

The following yoga study centers offer workshops and degree programs for serious yoga practitioners:

- **California Institute of Integral Studies:** A degree program for yoga studies in San Francisco. www.ciis.edu

- **Feathered Pipe Ranch:** Offers yoga-oriented workshops in Montana and the Caribbean. www.featheredpipe.com

- **Kripalu Center for Yoga and Health:** Offers yoga and fitness training in Lenox, Massachusetts. www.kripalu.org

- **Omega at the Crossings:** Offers yoga classes and workshops Austin, Texas. www.thecrossingsaustin.com

- **Omega Institute for Holistic Studies:** Offers retreats and workshops in California, New York, Florida, Costa Rica, and the Virgin Islands. www.eomega.org

- **Tassajara and Green Gulch Zen Centers:** Presents Zen and yoga instruction in San Francisco and Marin County. www.sfzc.org

Health, Yoga, and Fitness Organizations

The following organizations provide information to health and fitness professionals, including yoga teachers:

- **American Council on Exercise (ACE):** A nonprofit fitness certification and education provider. www.acefitness.org

- **ECA World Fitness:** Organization dedicated to furthering the education of health and fitness professionals. www.ecaworldfitness.com

- **IDEA Health & Fitness Association:** Membership organization of health and fitness professionals. www.ideafit.com

- **International Association of Yoga:** Membership association for yoga practitioners, teachers, therapists, and researchers. www.iayt.org

- **Yoga Alliance:** Support organization for yoga teachers. www.yoga alliance.org

- **Yoga Research and Education Center:** Studies the tradition, practices, and philosophy of yoga. www.yrec.org

Part VI
The Part of Tens

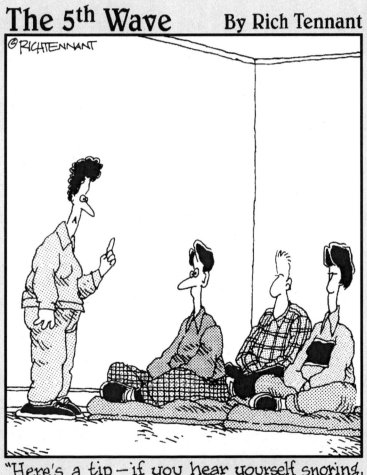

The 5th Wave   By Rich Tennant

"Here's a tip—if you hear yourself snoring, you're meditating too deeply."

In this part . . .

*E*very chapter in Part VI offers ten tidbits of good, rock-solid information. You find advice for getting motivated to do your yoga-with-weights workout, explanations of yoga-with-weights myths, and advice for charting your exercise progress.

You also find an appendix in this part that lists Web sites, magazines, books, and other goodies of interest to yoga-with-weights practitioners.

Index

346 **Yoga with Weights For Dummies**

• Y •

BUSINESS, CAREERS & PERSONAL FINANCE

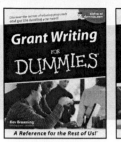

0-7645-5307-0

0-7645-5331-3 *†

Also available:
- ✔Accounting For Dummies †
  0-7645-5314-3
- ✔Business Plans Kit For Dummies †
  0-7645-5365-8
- ✔Cover Letters For Dummies
  0-7645-5224-4
- ✔Frugal Living For Dummies
  0-7645-5403-4
- ✔Leadership For Dummies
  0-7645-5176-0
- ✔Managing For Dummies
  0-7645-1771-6

- ✔Marketing For Dummies
  0-7645-5600-2
- ✔Personal Finance For Dummies *
  0-7645-2590-5
- ✔Project Management For Dummies
  0-7645-5283-X
- ✔Resumes For Dummies †
  0-7645-5471-9
- ✔Selling For Dummies
  0-7645-5363-1
- ✔Small Business Kit For Dummies *†
  0-7645-5093-4

HOME & BUSINESS COMPUTER BASICS

0-7645-4074-2

0-7645-3758-X

Also available:
- ✔ACT! 6 For Dummies
  0-7645-2645-6
- ✔iLife '04 All-in-One Desk Reference
  For Dummies
  0-7645-7347-0
- ✔iPAQ For Dummies
  0-7645-6769-1
- ✔Mac OS X Panther Timesaving
  Techniques For Dummies
  0-7645-5812-9
- ✔Macs For Dummies
  0-7645-5656-8

- ✔Microsoft Money 2004 For Dummies
  0-7645-4195-1
- ✔Office 2003 All-in-One Desk Reference
  For Dummies
  0-7645-3883-7
- ✔Outlook 2003 For Dummies
  0-7645-3759-8
- ✔PCs For Dummies
  0-7645-4074-2
- ✔TiVo For Dummies
  0-7645-6923-6
- ✔Upgrading and Fixing PCs For Dummies
  0-7645-1665-5
- ✔Windows XP Timesaving Techniques
  For Dummies
  0-7645-3748-2

FOOD, HOME, GARDEN, HOBBIES, MUSIC & PETS

0-7645-5295-3

0-7645-5232-5

Also available:
- ✔Bass Guitar For Dummies
  0-7645-2487-9
- ✔Diabetes Cookbook For Dummies
  0-7645-5230-9
- ✔Gardening For Dummies *
  0-7645-5130-2
- ✔Guitar For Dummies
  0-7645-5106-X
- ✔Holiday Decorating For Dummies
  0-7645-2570-0
- ✔Home Improvement All-in-One
  For Dummies
  0-7645-5680-0

- ✔Knitting For Dummies
  0-7645-5395-X
- ✔Piano For Dummies
  0-7645-5105-1
- ✔Puppies For Dummies
  0-7645-5255-4
- ✔Scrapbooking For Dummies
  0-7645-7208-3
- ✔Senior Dogs For Dummies
  0-7645-5818-8
- ✔Singing For Dummies
  0-7645-2475-5
- ✔30-Minute Meals For Dummies
  0-7645-2589-1

INTERNET & DIGITAL MEDIA

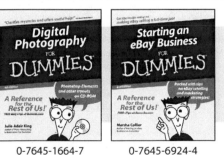

0-7645-1664-7

0-7645-6924-4

Also available:
- ✔2005 Online Shopping Directory
  For Dummies
  0-7645-7495-7
- ✔CD & DVD Recording For Dummies
  0-7645-5956-7
- ✔eBay For Dummies
  0-7645-5654-1
- ✔Fighting Spam For Dummies
  0-7645-5965-6
- ✔Genealogy Online For Dummies
  0-7645-5964-8
- ✔Google For Dummies
  0-7645-4420-9

- ✔Home Recording For Musicians
  For Dummies
  0-7645-1634-5
- ✔The Internet For Dummies
  0-7645-4173-0
- ✔iPod & iTunes For Dummies
  0-7645-7772-7
- ✔Preventing Identity Theft For Dummies
  0-7645-7336-5
- ✔Pro Tools All-in-One Desk Reference
  For Dummies
  0-7645-5714-9
- ✔Roxio Easy Media Creator For Dummies
  0-7645-7131-1

* Separate Canadian edition also available

† Separate U.K. edition also available

Available wherever books are sold. For more information or to order direct: U.S. customers visit www.dummies.com or call 1-877-762-2974.
U.K. customers visit www.wileyeurope.com or call 0800 243407. Canadian customers visit www.wiley.ca or call 1-800-567-4797.

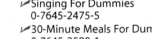

SPORTS, FITNESS, PARENTING, RELIGION & SPIRITUALITY

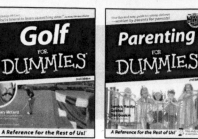

0-7645-5146-9

0-7645-5418-2

Also available:
- Adoption For Dummies
  0-7645-5488-3
- Basketball For Dummies
  0-7645-5248-1
- The Bible For Dummies
  0-7645-5296-1
- Buddhism For Dummies
  0-7645-5359-3
- Catholicism For Dummies
  0-7645-5391-7
- Hockey For Dummies
  0-7645-5228-7
- Judaism For Dummies
  0-7645-5299-6
- Martial Arts For Dummies
  0-7645-5358-5
- Pilates For Dummies
  0-7645-5397-6
- Religion For Dummies
  0-7645-5264-3
- Teaching Kids to Read For Dummies
  0-7645-4043-2
- Weight Training For Dummies
  0-7645-5168-X
- Yoga For Dummies
  0-7645-5117-5

TRAVEL

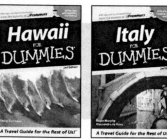

0-7645-5438-7

0-7645-5453-0

Also available:
- Alaska For Dummies
  0-7645-1761-9
- Arizona For Dummies
  0-7645-6938-4
- Cancún and the Yucatán For Dummies
  0-7645-2437-2
- Cruise Vacations For Dummies
  0-7645-6941-4
- Europe For Dummies
  0-7645-5456-5
- Ireland For Dummies
  0-7645-5455-7
- Las Vegas For Dummies
  0-7645-5448-4
- London For Dummies
  0-7645-4277-X
- New York City For Dummies
  0-7645-6945-7
- Paris For Dummies
  0-7645-5494-8
- RV Vacations For Dummies
  0-7645-5443-3
- Walt Disney World & Orlando For Dummies
  0-7645-6943-0

GRAPHICS, DESIGN & WEB DEVELOPMENT

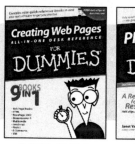
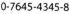
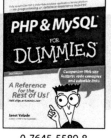

0-7645-4345-8

0-7645-5589-8

Also available:
- Adobe Acrobat 6 PDF For Dummies
  0-7645-3760-1
- Building a Web Site For Dummies
  0-7645-7144-3
- Dreamweaver MX 2004 For Dummies
  0-7645-4342-3
- FrontPage 2003 For Dummies
  0-7645-3882-9
- HTML 4 For Dummies
  0-7645-1995-6
- Illustrator CS For Dummies
  0-7645-4084-X
- Macromedia Flash MX 2004 For Dummies
  0-7645-4358-X
- Photoshop 7 All-in-One Desk
  Reference For Dummies
  0-7645-1667-1
- Photoshop CS Timesaving Techniques
  For Dummies
  0-7645-6782-9
- PHP 5 For Dummies
  0-7645-4166-8
- PowerPoint 2003 For Dummies
  0-7645-3908-6
- QuarkXPress 6 For Dummies
  0-7645-2593-X

NETWORKING, SECURITY, PROGRAMMING & DATABASES

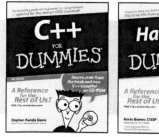
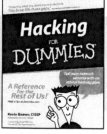

0-7645-6852-3

0-7645-5784-X

Also available:
- A+ Certification For Dummies
  0-7645-4187-0
- Access 2003 All-in-One Desk
  Reference For Dummies
  0-7645-3988-4
- Beginning Programming For Dummies
  0-7645-4997-9
- C For Dummies
  0-7645-7068-4
- Firewalls For Dummies
  0-7645-4048-3
- Home Networking For Dummies
  0-7645-42796
- Network Security For Dummies
  0-7645-1679-5
- Networking For Dummies
  0-7645-1677-9
- TCP/IP For Dummies
  0-7645-1760-0
- VBA For Dummies
  0-7645-3989-2
- Wireless All In-One Desk Reference
  For Dummies
  0-7645-7496-5
- Wireless Home Networking For Dummies
  0-7645-3910-8

HEALTH & SELF-HELP

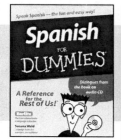

Diabetes FOR DUMMIES, 2nd Edition
0-7645-6820-5 *†

Low-Carb Dieting FOR DUMMIES
0-7645-2566-2

Also available:
- Alzheimer's For Dummies
  0-7645-3899-3
- Asthma For Dummies
  0-7645-4233-8
- Controlling Cholesterol For Dummies
  0-7645-5440-9
- Depression For Dummies
  0-7645-3900-0
- Dieting For Dummies
  0-7645-4149-8
- Fertility For Dummies
  0-7645-2549-2

- Fibromyalgia For Dummies
  0-7645-5441-7
- Improving Your Memory For Dummies
  0-7645-5435-2
- Pregnancy For Dummies †
  0-7645-4483-7
- Quitting Smoking For Dummies
  0-7645-2629-4
- Relationships For Dummies
  0-7645-5384-4
- Thyroid For Dummies
  0-7645-5385-2

EDUCATION, HISTORY, REFERENCE & TEST PREPARATION

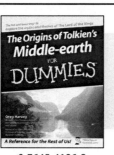

Spanish FOR DUMMIES
0-7645-5194-9

The Origins of Tolkien's Middle-earth FOR DUMMIES
0-7645-4186-2

Also available:
- Algebra For Dummies
  0-7645-5325-9
- British History For Dummies
  0-7645-7021-8
- Calculus For Dummies
  0-7645-2498-4
- English Grammar For Dummies
  0-7645-5322-4
- Forensics For Dummies
  0-7645-5580-4
- The GMAT For Dummies
  0-7645-5251-1
- Inglés Para Dummies
  0-7645-5427-1

- Italian For Dummies
  0-7645-5196-5
- Latin For Dummies
  0-7645-5431-X
- Lewis & Clark For Dummies
  0-7645-2545-X
- Research Papers For Dummies
  0-7645-5426-3
- The SAT I For Dummies
  0-7645-7193-1
- Science Fair Projects For Dummies
  0-7645-5460-3
- U.S. History For Dummies
  0-7645-5249-X

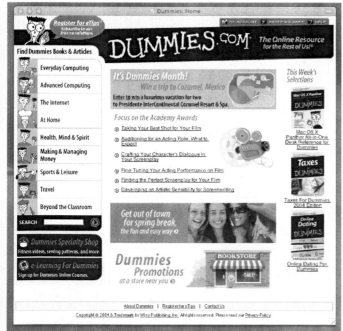

Get smart @ dummies.com®

- **Find a full list of Dummies titles**
- **Look into loads of FREE on-site articles**
- **Sign up for FREE eTips e-mailed to you weekly**
- **See what other products carry the Dummies name**
- **Shop directly from the Dummies bookstore**
- **Enter to win new prizes every month!**

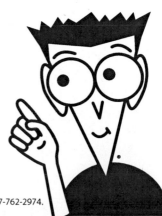

* Separate Canadian edition also available

† Separate U.K. edition also available

Available wherever books are sold. For more information or to order direct: U.S. customers visit www.dummies.com or call 1-877-762-2974.
U.K. customers visit www.wileyeurope.com or call 0800 243407. Canadian customers visit www.wiley.ca or call 1-800-567-4797.

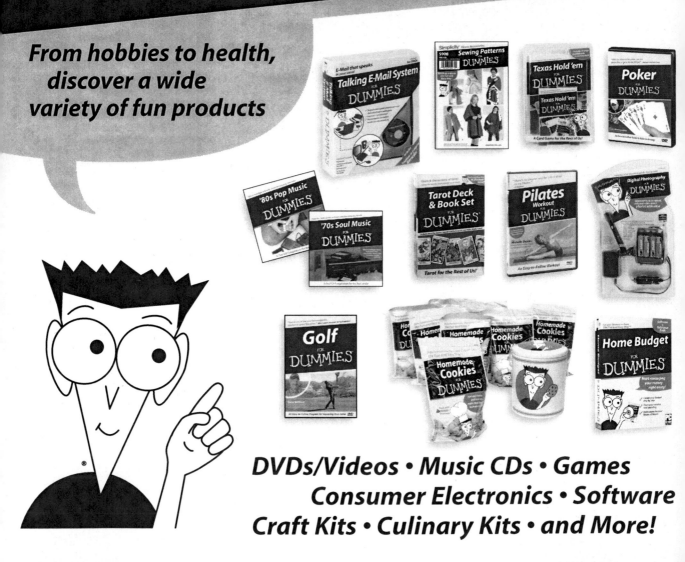
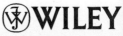

CPSIA information can be obtained at www.ICGtesting.com
Printed in the USA
BVOW01n0526030414

349558BV00007B/14/P